The Cambridge Psychological Library

COMMON PRINCIPLES
IN
PSYCHOLOGY & PHYSIOLOGY

COMMON PRINCIPLES
IN
PSYCHOLOGY & PHYSIOLOGY

by

JOHN T. MACCURDY

M.D. (Johns Hopkins), M.A. (Cantab.)

*Fellow of Corpus Christi College, and Lecturer in Psychopathology
in the University of Cambridge*

CAMBRIDGE

AT THE UNIVERSITY PRESS

1928

CAMBRIDGE
UNIVERSITY PRESS

University Printing House, Cambridge CB2 8BS, United Kingdom

Published in the United States of America by Cambridge University Press, New York

Cambridge University Press is part of the University of Cambridge.

It furthers the University's mission by disseminating knowledge in the pursuit of education, learning and research at the highest international levels of excellence.

www.cambridge.org
Information on this title: www.cambridge.org/9781107626164

© Cambridge University Press 1928

First published 1928
First paperback edition 2013

A catalogue record for this publication is available from the British Library

ISBN 978-1-107-62616-4 Paperback

Cambridge University Press has no responsibility for the persistence or accuracy of
URLs for external or third-party internet websites referred to in this publication,
and does not guarantee that any content on such websites is, or will remain, accurate
or appropriate.

To

W.S. & D.T.S.

CONTENTS

CONTENTS

PREFACE

IF we are to judge by the frequency with which the word is used, psychology is to-day one of the most popular of the sciences. A psychological novel, a psychological "fact" or a psychological experiment excites interest and respect. It might therefore be thought that psychology was a science deriving its authority from a theory, or group of theories, so widely accepted as to be virtually acknowledged as laws, that is as generalizations about mental phenomena carrying a high degree of predictability as to future phenomena or providing satisfactory explanations for a large number of otherwise uncorrelated mental happenings. A glance at psychological literature, however, would seem to suggest rather an opposite conclusion, namely that the popularity of psychology represented an acknowledgement of the importance of the study and a wish that it might have such a well-founded discipline.

In general biology we find the theory of evolution, variously interpreted perhaps, but nevertheless universally accepted. If we ask psychologists for their analogous, basic, psychological theory, however, we are offered (with equal confidence!) conditioned reflexes, *Gestalten*, unconscious sexuality, "purpose", glands of internal secretion, or "faculties". Each school has its facts, many of them unequivocal ones, and strongly in favour of the theory proposed: each, then, is probably expressing truth up to a certain point and not error. On the other hand, when general application is given to these theories, that is, when attempts are made to comprise all mental life in the formulae, irreconcilable differences of opinion arise. Two statements cannot both be true and yet conflict one with another. We must, therefore, assume either that the general explanations of only one of these schools are true or else that they are all inaccurate. In the former case, the true generalization which excludes the others must also eliminate the explanations for narrow groups of phenomena from which the rival generalizations were derived and which had seemed valid before being generalized. If this logical outcome were to be faced, we should have to deny, perhaps, that the behaviour of many animals at the breeding period was influenced by an endocrine cycle or, on the other hand, that children shewed "conditioned reflex" responses. The view that all the generalizations as yet achieved are inaccurate would seem to lead to less unhappiness and we are probably safe in adopting it.

If a basic psychological theory has yet to be framed, there may be two reasons for this. Either the phenomena considered by psychologists belong to categories that really are unrelated, or else they are related but the vocabulary useful in one category is useless in another. The latter seems the more promising view. and the primary object of this book is a suggested vocabulary, a vocabulary in which principles common to reflex action, to instincts and habits, to conscious and unconscious mental activities may be expressed.

In any discussion about nomenclature there is always some peacemaker who remarks with sententious finality that it does not matter what labels we use, what we want is facts! There is probably no more pernicious enemy of science than this man. It is undoubtedly true that a rose by any other name would 'smell as sweet (except to a suggestible subject!), but if the name is to have any classificatory or theoretic implication it is practically of as much importance for the development of science as is the phenomenon it labels. If we called a rose "beetroot", there would be an end of botany. This pacifist would probably have affirmed that it did not make any difference whether a chemist said that in combustion phlogiston was given off or oxygen added: combustion was combustion no matter in which terms it was described. Yet the simple translation of "addition or loss of phlogiston" into "loss or addition of oxygen" in the description of chemical actions paved the way for the development of modern chemistry. For most of the phenomena observed at the phlogistic period one was as good a formulation as the other; but the implications of the two vocabularies were momentous and opposed.

So long as scientific terms are words and not mere letters or numbers they are bound to carry some implication. In my present venture there is one implication that runs counter to current prejudice. In spite of the criticisms of the more philosophic biologists and physicists, the creed of the modern scientist is materialistic either in its formulations or tendency. That is, he looks avowedly for an explanation of all problems in terms of physico-chemical laws or else is trained to think only in such language and is thus unable to domesticate an alternative view. Yet, unfortunately, I am bound to propose a heresy. The principles which I detect, and hope to demonstrate, as common to mental behaviour of various types and to the physiology of the nervous system are immaterial agencies. If these were put into terms of physics and chemistry, the correlation, essential for any broad biological theory, would disappear. So I propose to assume that immaterial agencies, which I call patterns, do guide, and in that sense control, the physico-chemical processes involved in all living. Since the book is about patterns it would be foolish to explain them here but I may remark that their operation is analogous to the activity of the navigator who brings a vessel from port to port. Each single movement of the ship is adequately expressed and accounted for in mechanical terms but the voyage as a whole is the work of the navigator. In other words, the pattern theory is not a spiritistic one that assumes an appearance of energy from an extra-material sphere, but merely claims that exhibitions of energy in the biological field may be given their direction by agencies not subject to physico-chemical laws.

A preface is not the place for the exposition of the argument, but, rather, gives the author an opportunity of preparing the reader for what follows. Patterns represent properties and relations—pure abstractions—and yet I am gravely proposing to treat these abstractions as if they had some kind of existence apart from the material phenomena in which they are detected and as if they determined in some way the nature of these phenomena. This is a doctrine likely to meet with prejudice and is, at best, difficult to understand. It seems to fly in the face of common sense. Lest the reader should therefore discard it out of hand, it may be well to point out here that this is precisely the method and theory of mathematics, the utility of which cannot be gainsaid no matter what may be thought of its sanity.

In mathematics properties of number and relationship in time and space have been *abstracted* from the material phenomena in which they are displayed; these abstractions have then been dealt with as if they had an existence separable from their material representations. The combinations and interrelationships of number and dimension, possible and impossible, have been studied from the standpoint of logic (not as derived from experience) and in the end a system of laws, ever growing, has been erected that claims to have universal reference. The practical results of this method are better recognized popularly than is its "irrationality". In fact there lies in this discrepancy what is perhaps the most monstrous paradox of modern times. The contemporary citizen accepts as having material reality what can be shewn to follow mathematical laws, laws referring to relationships so abstract that they could exist if our material universe disappeared!

To the ordinary man the abstraction involved in using the formula "four times two is eight" is so habitual that he does not realize that he is invoking agencies that, although they are immaterial, regulate some of the properties of material objects. When, having counted the total number of cows in two lots of four each and found them to be eight, he predicts that two tricks of four cards each will contain eight cards altogether, he is unaware that what he has done is to abstract a property of a group of cows and apply it to a group of cards. To a hypothetical savage who cannot count this would appear as highly potent magic. The formula $4 \times 2 = 8$ seems rational to any of us, but when its method is put into non-numerical terms, it looks like madness— for what have cows to do with cards? Yet these terms do not misrepresent the method as the following example will shew, an example for which I am indebted to Professor G. I. Taylor.

He was anxious to learn about the distribution of stresses within a steel bar when it is twisted. For this he had an equation, but it was impossible to solve it using only mathematical symbols: some actual measurements were required. Obviously he could not measure anything within the steel bar without disturbing its structure. It happens, however, that the distortion under air pressure of a soap film stretched over a hole whose contour is the same as that of a cross-section of the bar could be expressed in the same equation as that for the distribution of strains within the bar. Now this soap bubble is available for measurement. So he measured the relative heights of such a bubble at various points and from this was able to tell what the strain would be at any point within the steel bar. Such a procedure flies right in the face of common sense. If proposed to a layman by one who was not a mathematician, it would be regarded as madness, for there is no similarity whatever between the physical properties of soap films and steel. To the non-mathematical it is as reasonable as weighing the ink used in drawing a picture of the bar in order to solve the above problem. To the mathematician, however, the physical properties of substances which give material representation of an equation are quite irrelevant. So long as the properties he is interested in are present, all others can be neglected just as we neglect the colour and habits of cows when counting the number of them in a herd.

In the light of the mathematical analogy, we are in a position to understand why it is expedient to discuss biological patterns in terms of the immaterial. Numbers we call digits because our forefathers counted on their fingers. Our children still begin their primitive arithmetic by counting fingers or other serial objects: this is the easiest way. But how far does it go? We quickly pass to simple generalizations about numbers and dimensions. Supposing we had to cling to their primitive material expressions in thinking about them, how cumbered we should be! If south were the position of the sun at noon, if horizontal meant a relationship to the horizon seen or imagined, if vertical were a position of balance in standing, how laboured our orientations would be! By generalization and abstraction we are emancipated from the material and thus gain control over it. But this control is limited to the range of the properties that are abstracted. Within the limit of finite numbers it is, humanly speaking, absolute. Six eggs added to six eggs will always make a dozen. Enough is known about electricity—another abstraction, by the way—for what used to appear only as a thunderbolt to become a slave of man. Less has been discovered about heredity, yet the breeder can produce some varieties with reasonable certainty. The behaviour of man is studied without reaching relevant abstractions, or, at least, these abstractions are not taken seriously, and so human behaviour is still sufficiently uncontrolled for both soldiers and pacifists to exist.

Mathematical abstractions, which are for the layman mostly mysteries, are accepted as impalpable and dealt with as abstractions. Mathematics have advanced because the laws governing the properties abstracted have been regarded as *sui generis*. A three-cornered sheet of iron has many properties. A geometrician treats it as a surface, then idealizes its shape, and with these two abstractions generalizes about triangles. The theorem that the three angles of a triangle together make two right angles holds for any flat surface and what the material may be that is co-extensive with the surface is irrelevant. On the other hand the metallurgist is indifferent to the shape of the sheet of iron but is interested in its texture, hardness, etc. He too, however, is able to put many of his abstractions into mathematical terms. But the worker with biological material finds relatively few phenomena that can be translated adequately into such language. In fact the arguments of the vitalist school as to the existence of non-material factors have never been answered except by citation from the materialistic creed. Whenever we meet with a process that is characteristic of living matter, we know it to be such from the very fact that it displays something unpredictable from the laws of Newtonian physics. These vital properties should be abstracted and treated as such. They then become, in my nomenclature, patterns—psychological, physiological, developmental and so on.

It appears to be obvious that, if patterns in the biological world could be formulated and their laws studied as mathematicians have done with those for number and dimension, biology would advance as have the physical sciences. This assumption, however, is probably not justified in the present stage of human mental development. The basic units with which the mathematician works are simple and stable. The biological sciences, on the other hand, are engaged in studying quality rather than quantity, something much more difficult to formulate. Moreover, since the essence of life is adaptation, the reactions of living matter are never stable: patterns are changing, slowly in the sphere of bodily form as exemplified in evolution, and rapidly in the sphere of behaviour. For these two reasons, he who tries to abstract the principles that underly and control living processes arrives at units that are neither simple nor stable: his task is, from the outset, more difficult than that of the mathematician. It is one that calls for a facility in dealing with abstractions such as the mathematician and the philosopher enjoy and, at the same time a familiarity with phenomena unknown to either of these savants.

These accomplishments are rarely combined so I cannot refrain from emphasizing that—apart from the facility or clumsiness of the style—any argument such as I am attempting is going to be followed easily only by those who are both sympathetic with its tendency and familiar with its mode of thought. How readers may vary in these two respects is shewn in the criticisms of the manuscript I have been privileged to receive from three scientists of note. The first is an unusually competent biologist. He complained that the general treatment was philosophic rather than strictly scientific; that he had difficulty in understanding my general position because he could not conceive of a pattern without a physical basis: "Because certain phenomena are *not yet* adequately explained on a mechanistic basis is no good reason for assuming that they are immaterial". In contrast was the point of view of a man recognized as an authority on the higher functions of the nervous system as revealed in both psychological and physiological investigation. He criticized the anti-mechanistic argument as being over elaborated because "I don't suppose any sane person thinks that 'mechanistic' theories, in our present state of knowledge, explain the phenomena". A middle position was assumed by one whose name is known in every anatomical and physiological laboratory the world around. He expressed himself as out of patience with the current materialistic assumptions because, he believed, they were sterilizing research. Yet he found my manuscript hard reading; this, he politely concluded, was due to his unfamiliarity with any type of thinking that was not materialistic in its subject matter. He wanted to think in terms of abstractions but found it arduous. For whom should I write? If these three learned men are typical, I have small hope of my presentation being wholly acceptable to any one and to many it may be intolerable.

Qui s'excuse s'accuse. I have been trying to explain why the reader is likely to make heavy weather in voyaging through the following pages and have written as if the difficulties lay wholly in the subject matter. This, however, is not the case and no one is more aware of it than myself. I suppose that everyone who speculates at all feels vastly inferior to his ideas. At least I know it to be true of myself. To realize that one has stumbled on formulae which, if applicable in one field, must hold for the whole territory of biology with equal validity (else the basic hypothesis is unsound), makes the discoverer sympathize with a mystic after his experience of universality: it is something he can neither describe nor understand himself. True abstractions in the present stage of human evolution defy clear formulation simply because they are abstract. It is the rarest of mortals who does not intuit, or "feel", abstractions rather than "know" them. For one who has had no philosophical training to claim that the importance of his theory is equalled by the lucidity of his style would be ὕβρις the enormity of which would shock him more than it could any Philistine critic. For my theory I will not apologize, but I do crave indulgence for the inadequacy of my expression.

If the reader's effort in following the argument be not intolerable, it is because I have been favoured with patient and painstaking criticism. For two successive years these formulations have been tried out in "lectures" to more advanced students of psychology in Cambridge. A lecture often consisted of five minutes of exposition and then fifty-five minutes of criticism and discussion. Under this fire unwarranted assumptions have been blown up, awkward facts reconciled, and hazy statements clarified. Foremost among the critics has been Mr F. C. Bartlett, for whose precision of attack I have as great a fear as I have gratitude for his patience and interest in attending the classes. I also owe much to two undergraduates, Mr Gregory Bateson and Mr R. W. Pickford, particularly the latter.

My debts are not fully acknowledged in recognizing these personal favours. In the present volume I am discussing problems successively in the fields of psychology, neurology and general biology. I cannot claim to be expert in any one of these subjects, for, as a specialist, I am only a psychiatrist. Consequently, my data are largely second-hand. Were it not for several classical works, the labour of gathering material, both relevant and accurate, would have exceeded my energy. Three of these must be mentioned specifically. First and foremost stands Sherrington's *Integrative Action of the Nervous System*, one of the monuments of modern physiology, distinguished alike for its originality, the soundness of its theory and the accuracy and wealth of the data recorded. In the field of animal behaviour I have drawn largely on the experiments of Koehler as described (so graphically) in his *Mentality of Apes*. Finally from Child's *The Origin and Development of the Nervous System* and *Physiological Foundation of Behaviour* I have found a key to much recent work in experimental biology and read a stimulating theory. These three authors have, of course, furnished introductions to literatures that have taken me far afield, but I have purposely reduced my references in the text so far as possible to books of this order. If it be desired to pursue reading in any of these fields, references will be found in the writings which are mentioned. The recently published work of Parsons, *An Introduction to the Theory of Perception*, can be warmly recommended as a guide to all the worth-while literature pertinent to the form and function of the nervous system.

Finally, a word should be added as to the general philosophic implications of my pattern theory. My education has never led me through the mazes of philosophy and I am as ignorant of its technical terms as I am unfamiliar with the habit of thought of the professed philosopher. Consequently, I am really incompetent to carry my generalizations beyond the range of the biological sciences, and for the few words in the last chapter in which a pattern metaphysic is suggested I beg the indulgence granted to a tyro. In particular, I must hasten to disavow any claim for proprietorship therein. It is quite possible that, when "patterns" are given universal reference, they merely repeat some well-known metaphysic. Specifically I suspect that Whitehead in the concluding chapters of his *Science and the Modern World* proposes a view that is analogous to, or identical with, what I am trying to express, but I am too innocent of mathematical philosophy to follow his argument with understanding. So I may be saying something quite different and should have no right to claim so great an authority as his in validation of my speculations.

J. T. M.

1928

PART ONE

PSYCHOLOGICAL PATTERNS

CHAPTER I

INTRODUCTION

IT is the purpose of this book to penetrate and, if possible, to destroy the bulkhead which has appeared between psychology and physiology, a partition that has created, artificially, two watertight compartments. It might be objected that the philosophy of materialism, which has so thoroughly permeated the thinking of cultured people in modern times, has long since broken down this barrier by making psychology a branch of biology, and biological data only a subdivision of physical phenomena. "During the epoch in question [nineteenth century], and indeed also at the present moment, the prestige of the more perfect scientific form belongs to the physical sciences. Accordingly, biology apes the manners of physics. It is orthodox to hold, that there is nothing in biology but what is physical mechanism under somewhat complex circumstances."[1] When we think "scientifically" we tell ourselves that thoughts are only epiphenomena, manifestations of underlying material activities and that "reality" belongs to the latter alone. This patter the layman cheerfully accepts from the science that has given him the internal combustion engine and wireless telephony. He says, so long as he is philosophizing, that the real world is composed of matter, stuff which reveals itself to his senses directly or indirectly. Thoughts have no existence apart from the words or signs which transmit them and the physiological processes which produce these expressions. His universe, as one protagonist of materialism puts it, is made up of atoms and aether; there is no room for ghosts. But this philosophy, although it relieves him of the necessity of going to church, has otherwise little effect on his daily life. Tacitly he constantly assumes the existence, the reality, the paramount importance of thoughts, even of those that evade and defy adequate expression. He allows the course of his life to be guided by ideals, entities no more material than the doctrine of the Trinity. And the orthodox

[1] A. N. Whitehead, *Science and the Modern World*, Cambridge, 1926.

scientist, when he leaves the laboratory or the rostrum, behaves in precisely the same way. Insensibly, therefore, we have drifted into a dualistic attitude. Our heads profess there is nothing but matter; in our hearts we know mind exists. Say what we will, the bulkhead holds, the watertight compartments are there.

The point of this preamble is that it is not a simple task to do away with this dissociation. Experience seems to shew us that there are two separate worlds; and that this judgment is more emotional than intellectual makes it the more inexpugnable. The reader, then, is almost certainly prejudiced in advance and will, therefore, have a hard time to understand the argument. Added to his task will probably be a necessity to lay aside his materialistic bias that—willy-nilly—has become part of the mental fabric of every civilized man to-day. To quote Whitehead again: "We are now so used to the materialistic way of looking at things, which has been rooted in our literature by the genius of the seventeenth century, that it is with some difficulty that we understand the possibility of another mode of approach". Finally, there is a technical difficulty, well-nigh insurmountable. Even if what I hope to shew be granted, that psychological and physiological phenomena are the expressions of the same underlying agencies, the fact remains that the phenomena are different, they are labelled with different terms and studied by different methods. Most important of all, they are investigated by different men. Hence the psychologist is rarely conversant with physiology and *vice versa*. A vocabulary applicable to either field is bound to be foreign to workers in both subjects. To have the argument skip from one field to the other is certain to be puzzling and I will try to avoid it so far as possible. If the reader is to remain unconfused, he must bear in mind the general programme of the book and keep himself constantly oriented thereby. My first task is, therefore, to sketch out the argument.

In an effort to understand emotions I have brought together and analysed a rather large number of observations drawn mainly from psychopathological material, since, in this, emotional reactions are relatively more prominent than in normal life.[1] The conclusion was reached that emotions appear when instinctive responses are stimulated but do not reach untrammelled expression. This led naturally to an examination of the nature of "instinct",

[1] *Psychology of Emotion Morbid and Normal*, London, Kegan Paul, 1925.

which was found to be an automatic, unreflective type of habit reaction, the habit being either racial or individual in origin. In other words, this "instinct" may be looked on as a set behaviour pattern, modified perhaps by consciousness, but never initiated thereby. Examination of mental life from the genetic and objective points of view, which has been fostered by both psychopathology and behaviourism, has produced the modern theory that the basic structure of mind is to be found in such patterns, and many behaviourists go so far as to claim that the superstructure is similarly composed. That is, psychology can get along without the concepts of consciousness and will. For centuries our infant science has been swaddled in wrappings of metaphysics and epistemology, its individuality hidden and its growth prevented. If it is to have a chance to develop, these garments or bandages must be removed. The behaviourists seem to have thrown the baby out with the bath, but that does not mean a change was undesirable. The formula as applicable to the foundations of mental life would seem to be useful. At least, to me it appears so fruitful an hypothesis that I am taking it as the starting point of the present work.

One of its chief advantages is that it makes unnecessary any sharp discrimination between the physiological and the psychological. A "pattern" can refer equally well to integrated reflexes and to instincts. And nowhere is this more valuable than in dealing with emotions where bodily manifestations play such an obvious rôle. The James-Lange hypothesis would claim that what is subjectively felt is just the somatic disturbance. Unfortunately, this admirably simple formula is rendered untenable in its original statement by the findings of neurology, both experimental and clinical. Emotions, exhibited both objectively and subjectively, may persist when practically all of the body is cut off from nervous connection with the brain. To get round this difficulty Lloyd Morgan and Sherrington have proposed that visceral reactions may have some sort of re-presentation in the cerebral cortex which is capable of reactivation. This assumption makes possible the correlation of a large number of phenomena and I have adopted it, calling these "re-presentations", for reasons to be discussed shortly, "images". Such "images", I hope to shew, form an integral part of reaction patterns, which are, indeed, nothing but sequences of images that serve as stimuli for separate elements in a train of actions, in the absence of present, material stimuli appropriate for such actions. A general and tentative conclusion from the study of emotions was that *the basis of mental life is an unconscious flux of images; when these enter consciousness, becoming subjective data, they are the fundamental elements of which "thoughts" are composed; on the other hand, they initiate and control many physiological processes of both voluntary and involuntary systems.* The present work is to be devoted to the elucidation and development of this formula.

First, I shall review the conclusions cited above, outlining the nature of the evidence on which they were based, and from this go on to study the way in which consciousness utilizes the unconscious flux of images to produce the different kinds of mental events which have been called faculties. This will lead to the formulation of certain Laws of Patterns as exhibited in the mental field.

Second will come an excursion into the realm of physiology. To call the basis of mental life the higher functions of the nervous system is the crassest kind of tautology. I shall try, rather, to shew that the reaction pattern is composed of a flux of "images" which appear first in quite simple physiological processes. If past experience operates in the present without a material reappearance, something of the nature of "image" is in existence. If this repetition occurs at a primitive physiological level, then something, which is ordinarily held to be peculiar to mind, is characteristic of so-called non-mental activities as well. In fact, I shall go so far as to claim that this reappearance of the past in the present is what differentiates organic from inorganic nature. I would suggest that the relationship between physiologic and psychologic is not merely one of analogy but of an identity of an essential element common to both. This is, of course, like the materialistic claim, but according to my scheme the identity resides in an element that is impalpable, immaterial, the very "stuff that dreams are made on."

In order to make clear this point and to lay the ghost of materialism, I may borrow an analogy invented by Dr Clark-Kennedy to explain to his medical students the mysteries of physiology. Suppose some inhabitants of Mars descend to our earth and investigate a railway train and its behaviour. These Martians know all about Newtonian physics, the laws of thermodynamics and so on. They have the same senses as we, but, we presume, cannot perceive human beings directly; and—to avoid Gilbertian embarrassments—to them human raiment and tools are also imperceptible. The creatures set themselves to study a passenger train. It is seen at once that the engine pulls and the brakes stop it. Elaborate measurements and calculations shew that consumption of coal meets all the energy requirements, the locomotive and brakes are analysed and comprehended, the law of the conservation of energy holds. But why does it progress by fits and starts? What makes the throttle open or close? This unseen agency troubles the materialistic Martian until some intrepid experimenter puts his hand on the appropriate levers and finds that he can start and stop the train as well as any ghost. The Martians now use the trains and the theory of ghosts is remembered only as a superstition of unenlightened days. It is true that there are mischievous sceptics who will keep pointing out that no one has yet explained why luggage will insist on passing from the platform to the train or *vice versa*. But the mass and inertia of the luggage are so trifling when compared with that of the train and the quantity of it varies so much that it is evident to common sense that luggage has nothing whatever to do with the running of the train. Besides it is an interesting example of a tropism! And then one day some idle Martian strays by a football field and observes the extraordinary movements of the ball. When his report has been accepted and his observations confirmed, consternation rules until some savant shews that in all its long parabolic flights known ballistic principles are in operation. The principle of the conservation of energy holds! Some heretics continue sceptical, however, and they revert to the study of trains. They assume that there are ghosts, because nothing but ghosts could account for so many of the football's movements. In order to discover the habits of these ghosts, correlated mysteries are scrutinized. It is learned that cabs, 'buses and lorries come to the stations and depart in a definite time relation to the trains. The passenger vehicles are a puzzle, but the goods in the lorries can be followed. The latter lead to farms, factories and warehouses. The economic life of man is reconstructed from the behaviour of his goods. Eventually, even the rules of his games and religions are sketched out. The life of man is known; but he himself remains an hypothesis. It is important to note, however, that the more is found out about this hypothetical man, the more his body can be reconstructed, the fewer do the exceptions to the law of the conservation of energy become. "Man" is an answer to the Martian's question "Why", not to "How". In any competent theory purpose and mechanism explain each other mutually; they should never be mutually exclusive.

If the argument of this analogy be now applied to biological study, the programme I have set myself may be more readily understood. Mechanism explains so much in the field of physiology that it distracts attention from the problem of purpose. When we turn to psychology, however, mechanism explains little or degenerates into tautology. On the other hand, psychology is characterized by purpose, a view that William McDougall has so skilfully popularized. But so soon as "purpose" is identified in simpler mental reactions, it begins to be detectable in physiological phenomena as well. There is—from a materialistic standpoint—some unknown factor or factors running through the whole of life, no matter how vital activity may be expressing itself. The natural field wherein to investigate this X is that in which it is most prominent. So, if we wish to discover the laws of what is non-mechanical, we should study the phenomena least complicated by mechanism, that is to say, the mental. Having worked out these laws, we may then turn to physiology and see whether the psychological laws in their simplest forms cover the X at that biological level as well. The second part of this book will, then, be devoted to an attempted answer of physiological questions in terms that were originally psychological. If the endeavour succeed, we shall have got a vocabulary that is at once psychological and physiological, in other words that is truly biological. Essentially, I am not trying to answer fundamental questions, but to provide a terminology in which they may be discussed without prejudice.

CHAPTER II

DEFINITIONS OF "IMAGES"

As stated in the last chapter, a conclusion from the study of emotions was that these arise when instinctive processes are activated but do not achieve immediate or free expression. We must now consider what some of these terms mean and what the statement implies.

For present purposes an instinct may be taken to be a pattern of behaviour; that is a set, routine, automatic mode of response to a given stimulus. When this pattern is in free operation, a series of co-ordinated muscular movements takes place, and—so the evidence seems to indicate—nothing else occurs. If, however, the reaction is held up in any way, then a kind of overflow appears which constitutes emotion. This in turn may be exhibited in two ways, emotional expression and affect. The former consists of contractions of voluntary limb muscles in gestures, of face muscles in grimacing, smiling, etc., and of various integumental and visceral discharges (sweat secretion, hair erection, changes in blood pressure, contraction of the walls of hollow viscera, endocrine secretions and so on). The biological origin and function of these emotional expressions has been studied by many workers, from Darwin onward. Affect is the peculiarly subjective and personal reaction that conscious beings experience with emotions, it is "feeling".

There are large problems involved in the answer to the question as to what physiological and psychological processes underlie this strange phenomenon of affect. My conclusion has been that, although bodily changes may—and undoubtedly do—produce an effect on consciousness as a vague and unlocalizable "feeling", unconscious mental disturbances play an important, and perhaps dominant, rôle. What is the nature of these latter activities? Morton Prince has hypnotized patients suffering from attacks of distressing affect and then got a retrospective account of painful experiences going on at the time of an attack, described as anyone will retail a vivid dream of the night before. At the time of the attack the patient is consciously quite unaware of these mental processes. Since these dream-like experiences take the form in memory of images (as indeed most true dreams do) and since they are active although not at the time conscious, Prince has called them "co-conscious" images. In my book on Emotion I have given considerable space to a discussion of such phenomena and have even suggested that in such co-conscious images we may find the roots for all our conscious thoughts and actions. But, before we can go on to a consideration of this hypothesis, it is necessary to consider a basic question. What is an image? How can something that we know only as a consciously introspected phenomenon be justifiably conceived as existing unconsciously?

One would expect to see "image" defined in every text-book of psychology, but I was surprised to find the meaning taken for granted in five standard text-books in which I searched. The nearest approach I could discover was this sentence from William James: "Sensations, once experienced, modify the nervous organism, so that copies of them arise again in the mind after the original outward stimulus is gone". This occurs in his *Principles* at the beginning of the chapter on Imagination; perhaps it is intended as a definition. In a more recent book Woodworth[1] gives a definition: "A sensation or complex of sensations recalled by a substitute stimulus is called a 'mental image' or a 'memory image'".

Etymologically the word image is derived from the same root as gives *imitation*. So the notion of repetition, echoing, copying, is there. But it is not an exact, complete repetition, for, if it were, the phenomena of hallucination would occur: there must be some kind of dilution or weakening in the reproduction. Plainly our definition must introduce some discrimination between the normal and abnormal types of reproduction of past experience.

Again, is consciousness necessarily present when true images appear? When a patient describes a scene enacted before his eyes that would account adequately for his reaction, are we to deny an imaginal form to these mental processes because the subject was unaware of them at the time, merely in that part of his whole mental structure which we call consciousness? Or the argument may be brought nearer home, brought within the experience of quite normal people. When we sleep we are not conscious, at

[1] Robert S. Woodworth, *Psychology, A Study of Mental Life.*

least not in the ordinary sense of that term. But on waking we may recall experiences that we know were not the product of external stimuli; they seem to be indubitable reproductions of past sensory impressions and—retrospectively at least—quite vivid ones. The normal remembering of a dream is, then, analogous to, if not identical with, the retrospection by the hypnotized patient of his co-conscious images. If images (like some other data of consciousness) are to be admitted as existing only when registered by an active subjective awareness, a good deal of important psychological material is going to be neglected. It would even be possible to use this criterion relentlessly and arrive at the logical, solipsistic conclusion that I alone know what an image is! Indeed, if an introspective psychology sticks rigorously and honestly to its own chosen field, this kind of sterility is inevitable. If it surreptitiously uses objective data, it does so clumsily, for it has neither the vocabulary nor the formulae with which to handle them. It is only since psychology has avowedly adopted the objective method that it has gained the right to group itself with the biological sciences.

If we are to bring imaginal processes within the sway of the objective method we must have a definition of image in terms of behaviour. When I am subjectively aware of a discrete bit of past sensory experience *I* know that I have an image thereof. If I remain motionless and silent, no one else can tell what my mental content is. But, on the other hand, I may behave *as if* a specific, past stimulus were now in operation. If I cower when confronted by a man who has previously beaten me, an onlooker would say that I imagined I was going to be beaten again. Here there is some kind of reproduction of past experience and, therefore, we will say that some kind of imaginal process is in operation. But it would be unwise to jump to the conclusion that I have a true image, unless we are ready to rob that term of all its specificity. The observer does not know whether my mental content is of an abstract thought of physical suffering, whether I actually believe that my opponent is now raising his hand to strike, whether I am visualizing an ordeal knowing it to be only a memory, or, indeed, whether I am aware of anything—I may not even realize that I am making shrinking movements. All he knows is that I am not at the moment threatened, but that I am behaving as if I were. This kind of reproduction of past experience which is betrayed solely by behaviour we will call "image function". It may affect consciousness as a true image, or it may remain wholly unconscious; the use of the term image function implies nothing whatever as to the presence or absence of introspective awareness. It is something known only by its effects: it is, so to speak, a stimulus that is not materially present.

An image function, if it take the form of a mental presentation and becomes an introspected datum, may be either a true image or an hallucination. It would carry us too far afield to attempt at this point to discover the method we use when we make a subjective discrimination between the two. Now it is important to gather objective criteria for differentiation. In the layman's terms, a person who experiences an image is thinking of something that is not there, while, if he hallucinates, he is seeing, hearing, something that is not there. Why does the layman judge of one person that he is in a reverie or cogitating while of another that he is delirious? The opinion is reached without a shred of intro-spective evidence, but it is held confidently. Plainly, then, the behaviour resulting from images and hallucinations must be dif-ferent. A simple example will shew that the former excites an indirect, the latter a direct, response. If I am hungry and hallu-cinate some food, I pick up the imaginary food and put it into my mouth, even—if the hallucination continues—going so far as to chew and swallow it. On the other hand, if hunger leads to an image of food, I begin at once to image the place where it is and the road thither. If I follow the dictates of appetite, I actually go to the cupboard and eat actual food. (With many people, of course, the preliminary planning would be carried out more in "thoughts" than in images, but I happen to be enough of a visualist for this description to be literally true.) So an hallucination leads to a direct and simple response appropriate to the nature of the stimulus which is reproduced, while the image evokes other images with such of the responses appropriate to the latter as to build up a programme of action having as its goal the experiencing in actuality of the stimulus represented originally as the first image of the series. If the primary image excites no overt behaviour, an ob-server is, of course, in total ignorance of there being any image at all; but even elementary introspection teaches us that, in any reverie, this programme is carried out in imagination. In other words, everyday experience teaches us that images do not remain, unchanging and permanently isolated in consciousness: their normal result is more images and the evocation of indirect and associated reactions, but not an immediate response appropriate to the nature of the primary image.

This would seem to justify an important generalization: that a function of images is to reproduce elements of past experience and *combine* them into programmes, plans or fantasies, of action. Images serve as links in a chain of associated mental processes.

The human adult with his highly specialized intelligence can effect these combinations with ease provided they be not too complicated. But when "learning" is necessary, another kind of imaginal process can be discerned. Let us consider a simple example. I am being taught a string of unrelated words. After hearing them once I may be able to repeat the first two or three, but no effort will resuscitate memory of the others. Sufficient repetition will, however, enable me to repeat the whole list accurately. Between this final capacity and the beginning point where any given word seems totally strange and senseless to me, there are stages where the word is first familiar on its being repeated by my teacher, and then where I can summon the word myself if given the first letter or syllable. Past experience, in these stages, is doing something. But it is not an image, for I am not conscious of it. Nor is it an image function, as that term has so far been defined, for it is producing no reaction—by itself—that can be detected either subjectively or objectively. The reproduction seems to be present only in some incomplete form. What would have been an incomplete stimulus in the first instance will now, however, produce the completed image or image function. Let us suppose that the word in question is "beware" and the one before it in the list, "duty". Provided there is no pre-existent association in my mind between these words, nothing but the clear enunciation of the whole word will bring "beware" into consciousness at the beginning of the experiment. After a few repetitions, the syllable "be-" will produce the response "beware". Later, the initial letter will do it, or even my seeing the lips of my teacher coming together as if to form a labial consonant. Finally the word "duty" alone, acting as an audible stimulus or merely imaginally, will lead to the reproduction of "beware". In this series, a continually smaller and smaller representation of the stimulus has served to evoke the reaction, until finally the original stimulus is not represented at all.

At this point, there is a complete image, or image function, and we know that it is an image *because* what occasions its appearance is not a representation of the stimulus at all but merely an association that has been formed with an earlier response. In other words, the threshold for the stimulus has gradually fallen until it has become zero. Before the process of reproducing a bit of past experience has been completed, traces of the reproduced impression will shew themselves in a lowering of threshold for a repetition of the original response. Such an incomplete image, or image function, I shall call a *liminal image*.

Our final definition to cover true images, image functions and liminal images will be: *An imaginal process, from the standpoint of an objective observer, is some kind of a reproduction of a specific bit of past sensory experience, which is inferred to exist from the presence of a reaction for which the specific experience would be the appropriate stimulus—this reaction not being completely accounted for by any demonstrable environmental event.*

A moment's consideration will shew that, by eliminating introspection as a necessary or essential element, we have arrived at a definition of something which might appear in conscious, unconscious, or even physiological reactions. It would be present whenever an organism—or even an organ—shews a modification of behaviour by experience such that it seems as if it "remembered" the experience. In this concept there is, of course, nothing wholly new. Biology has long since recognized the principle of organisms being modified by experience in behaviour and even in form. Essentially the same principle has been labelled *Bahnung* (literally, "pathway-making," but often translated "facilitation") by Exner, *Associative Memory* by Loeb, *Engraphy* by Semon, or *Conditioning* by Pavlov. The one novelty in the formulation I am proposing is the adoption of a psychological terminology for something that has a wide biological reference. Superficially, it may seem as if my "imaginal process" is identical with Semon's "mneme", for in both doctrines a far-reaching theory is based on the vital capacity of registration and re-activation of experience. Semon's theory is, however, materialistic in its tendency, while mine is just the reverse. The impress of experience, according to Semon, is some kind of a physical alteration of protoplasm, an effect, too subtle perhaps for demonstration with present-day technique and, therefore, known only by its modification of function, but nevertheless a material change. He says of an *engram* (p. 24),[1] "It would be a mistake...to use a term like 'memory image', which invariably suggests phenomena in consciousness". It is for this very reason that I have chosen to speak of imaginal processes. I wish to stress the immateriality of the phenomenon and have, therefore, chosen a term which will imply—if implication there must be—something immaterial, for we all tend, intuitively, to regard thoughts as belonging to a different category from those data which impress us *via* extrospection. A label for the process that will suggest something psychological is therefore desirable if it will facilitate an understanding of my thesis that the data of introspection are only the highly elaborated and complicated products of an immaterial something, which first appears as a mere modifiability of reaction in lowly organisms, but which at the end of its evolution is known not merely as conscious images but even as thoughts. It is significant that to exemplify an "engram" Semon begins with purely psychological phenomena.

Semon has systematized his views in both the biological and psychological fields with his doctrine of the *mneme*, the "memory" of living tissues. According to this theory, experience is written into protoplasm as an *engram*, from which it may be re-activated or *ecphorized*, as he says. He thus ascribes to bodily events a process ordinarily regarded as something peculiar to mental life alone. Memory, or at least its generalized biological form of "mneme", becomes a phenomenon of all living matter, that we detect most easily in the operation of our minds, merely because it reaches its more obvious and facile expression there. With this I most heartily agree; in fact this doctrine may have been, unconsciously, an important factor in the genesis of my hypotheses although I had only heard of, and not read, Semon's work when I first formulated my general scheme.

On the other hand, Semon's theory fails, in my opinion, of its potential usefulness because of an unfortunate inconsistency in its development. The engram is held to be some kind of an effect in protoplasm, too subtle for demonstration with present day technique, but, nevertheless, a physical something. The mneme and memory are thus reduced, fundamentally, to physico-chemical phenomena: physico-chemical laws, it is believed, will somehow, sometime, be shewn to be the principles by which inert matter produces the highest and most impalpable products of biological activity. In the end, mechanism is invoked as the fundamental agency, the apparent heresy against the modern religion of materialism is explained away: Semon is, after all, orthodox.

[1] Richard Semon, *The Mneme*, London, Allen and Unwin, 1921. Semon's work is largely an elaboration of theories put forward by Hering and Samuel Butler.

This is an excellent example of the miracles which faith can perform in surmounting the judgments of common sense, the judgments derived by simple observation and obvious deduction therefrom. We laugh at the savage who fears that his enemy will annihilate him by destroying parings from his finger nails. The idea of making a Shakespeare sonnet in a test tube ought to seem equally ludicrous. Both are instances of magic, that is the production of effects not predictable, nor thinkable, as a result of the manipulation of the materials used which operate according to the known laws of the properties of those materials. It is legitimate to imagine the development of television through the application of known physical laws; but it is not legitimate to expect a Rutherford to produce Monna Lisas or Sistine Madonnas in his laboratory. The best he could do would be to copy them with absolute accuracy. The materials used in the production of a beautiful object are constituted in accordance with mechanical principles and may be studied in a laboratory, but the beauty is a product of the arrangement of these elements, an arrangement which is quite independent of the physico-chemical processes which have brought the elements into being. The laws, or rules or canons, which govern this arrangement, are those of aesthetics, not of mechanics: so aesthetics and mechanics cannot be correlated, nor the laws of one category utilized to produce effects in the other. Values, of any human order, belong to a different category from that comprising phenomena that engage the workers in laboratories. If one analyses values, a process which is purely psychological, the factors that emerge remain permanently in the mental, or at least biological, sphere and never become physical except by an act of faith, similar to that of Semon's.

I have chosen an example of aesthetic values because the chasm which separates them from phenomena in the material world is too wide to be bridged by any structure beginning on the latter side. An attempt to translate the beauty of a picture into mechanical terms could only result in a formula of such clumsiness that its tautology would be obvious to the least philosophically minded. When we turn, however, to such mental events as correlate reactions to physical phenomena, it is possible to fabricate a formula in terms of the physiology of reflexes and so on, in which so many clear facts are stated as to make the tautology less glaring. This is what the behaviourists have achieved. They account for the reactions of a man in terms of bodily processes, much as an engineer might account for the movements of an ocean liner, each and every one of which is explicable by physical laws. The sum total of these movements brings the vessel from port to port. Therefore, says the behaviourist-engineer, the voyage is wholly explained as a sum of these units: the ship sails itself across the ocean. Each statement to the conclusion is easily shewn to be true, but the common man knows the deduction to be false, not because he detects a logical fallacy, but because he knows that a navigator is essential. Some one has to plan the way the unit movements are to be put together before the vessel could ever reach port.

Mechanistic physiologists and mechanistic biologists argue in the same way about the reactions of living organisms. In this case, the units, that are adequately expressed in physico-chemical terms, are not so well known nor calculable as in the case of the ship. The mechanist, however, his hope buoyed up by the discovery of the physico-chemical factors involved in more and more of the units, assumes that in the future they may all be determined and that then life will be translatable into terms of physics and chemistry. Like the behaviourists they fail to see that no conceivable increase of knowledge along these lines could explain the design or plan which unites them into a working whole. This failure causes them little discomfort because their working hypothesis is in accord with their religion—materialism; and they feel themselves logically unassailable until every unit problem is solved in materialistic terms and the riddle still unanswered. An argument based on what *may* be found is hard to rebut.

I have indulged in this excursion in order to shew why Semon's "mneme" is theoretically sterile. He invokes what I am convinced is a useful principle, but short-circuits his argument when he makes of the "engram" a protoplasmic alteration in the first instance.

CHAPTER III

"PATTERNS"

MENTAL activities, as revealed to introspection, are so rich, varied and kaleidoscopic that the mere cataloguing of them seems a task impossible to achieve with finality. The different "faculties" have shifting boundaries, and it is always open to a psychologist to eliminate any one of them by describing its phenomena in terms of others. For instance, is there, or is there not, such a thing as "free will"? Such a question is never answered satisfactorily in terms of his specialty by the introspective psychologist for two interconnected reasons. In the first place, the animus is philosophical rather than psychological, for whole systems of metaphysics stand or fall by the answer. Secondly, the data invoked to establish or repudiate the claim are subjective, not objective. If this antithesis means anything at all, it must imply at least a danger of preferential selection of subjective data. The one hope of psychology as a science rests on the possibility of analysis revealing simpler, less varying, mental elements, acting as a foundation on which the multiform superstructure known to introspection rests, and recurring with sufficient regularity to justify use of them in classification.

An analogy may make this point clearer. Functions superficially inconspicuous but of fundamental importance are performed in the same way and effected through similar organs in all mammalia. Zoologists use these data in a classification that is satisfactory scientifically because it is objective. In earlier days, when subjective criteria preponderated, the barnacle goose was classed as "fish". In observation of the subjective type, human interests and human symbolical valuations determined the selection of what was to be seen. Now the camel, bat, whale, tiger and man are all classed together as mammals, a grouping which affronts common sense. Common sense deals with things as they obviously are and spurns subtleties; so the bat is a bird, or the whale is a fish, even to such an accomplished observer as Herman Melville.

But the analyses of comparative anatomists, embryologists and physiologists all reveal the same general plan on which the basic functions of circulation, respiration, digestion, excretion and reproduction are both built and operated in the class Mammalia. The pertinence of the analogy lies in the fact that the general plan is not revealed to naïve common sense, a recognition of it does not grant the layman any symbolic satisfaction and it may even be detrimental to his economic adaptations; the plan, moreover, is not directly observable, it is not even a material thing, but an abstraction, like the idea in the mind of an architect when he sketches the design of a new building. Yet it is universally accepted by biologists for these very reasons. Because it is an abstraction and because it neglects the obvious, it gives the biologist a means of ignoring differences which are of paramount importance to the layman. In other words, it enables him to be objective and to eliminate subjective criteria. It manufactures a set of scientific values. Subjectively, he is ruled by a set of values derived from the needs of everyday human adaptation. For a student of nature, the human standard is irrelevant and even misleading. The scientist, then, is prepared if necessary to ignore the obvious and spurn common sense, when he becomes objective. This does not mean that he is blind, that he fails to observe that the whale is bigger than the mouse and that it does not walk on the ground. But size-scale and habitat are irrelevant to the purpose in hand, so he neglects them, although, subjectively and as a mere man, they impress him much more than does the embryonic, skeletal structure of these animals.

We are looking for simple mental elements that may serve as building blocks in the foundation supporting the superstructure known to consciousness. It has already been suggested that the elements required may be imaginal processes. If so, the question arises, What are the means whereby they are united, arranged, or grouped? The answer is, *Patterns*. Before going on to describe them—for indeed the whole of this book is an attempt to do so—it may be well to relate how this notion of mental patterns has arisen.

As has been mentioned in the first chapter, the conclusion was reached from a study of emotions that these reactions are determined by underlying "instinctive" processes, activated but not reaching complete expression in their natural bodily movements. It is the boiling-over, so to speak, of the heated instinct, which provides the "push" of the emotion. To follow the metaphor, the liquid—instinct—is turned into steam, which is the emotion. But there are many different kinds of emotional expressions and myriads of shades of feeling. The nature or quality of the emotion seems to depend on the nature of the instinctive processes that are co-consciously active at the moment. Co-conscious thoughts are not, by definition, available for direct examination, but their nature may be inferred from coincident action and speech, or special psychological technique may induce a retrospective delineation of them. An investigation of emotions would, therefore, have been incomplete, had it not included some exploration of the unconscious, concomitant activities, and some speculation as to the nature of unconscious mental processes. It would be inappropriate to rehearse the observations that are recorded *in extenso* in my book on Emotion, or to repeat all the arguments there used in a hypothetical reconstruction of the activities underlying them. It is sufficient for our present purposes to indicate these and state conclusions.

All the available evidence seems to point to the conclusion that the less consciousness is active, the less attention is being consistently oriented to some specific internal or external situation, the more random and lawless does thinking become. That is, the less do the laws of association, as derived from introspection, seem to hold. But when we say that anything is lawless or irrational, we are merely admitting our ignorance of the laws that are in operation, or else abandoning the working hypothesis of all science that Nature always works according to law, that every event is preceded by a cause. Freud's greatest gift to psychology is probably his theory of free associations, because intrinsic therein is his "unconscious", which rationalizes not only the symptoms of the psychoneurotic and psychotic, but also the innumerable irrationalities of healthy people. Since many psychologists seem loath to see anything new in Freud's doctrine of free associations, it may be well to explain what the differences are between consciously regulated and free associations, or, to use Jung's terms, between directed and undirected thinking.

In directed thinking, we employ associations that are logical. That is, the relationship between the entities that are brought together is one of coincidence or sequence in space or time, expresses cause and effect, or some part-whole connection. Examples of such associations are: chair—table, Maundy Thursday—Good Friday, water-fall—power, arc—circle. The relationships between these pairs are so obvious that the naturalness of their conjunction is apparent to anyone. In other words, it is inherent in the entities themselves, and does not require a sentence to explain why they are brought together. If the words used did not call up these, and similar, associations immediately, they would be meaningless. The utility of speech is dependent on them: they are adaptive for all who speak the language. They appeal to universal experience.

On the other hand, experience that is esoteric may lie behind associations that are adaptive. To understand the reason for the connection between the elements that are thus brought together, it is necessary to have familiarity with the background experience. For instance, "Mays"—River is meaningful to some thousands who know that the inter-college rowing races held in the May Term at Cambridge are called "The Mays". But the pair of words would be nonsense to most Americans, indeed it would probably be heard as "Maze River".

Finally, the background experience may be purely individual and the association, therefore, quite senseless to all but the subject. But it may nevertheless be quite adaptive. If I wish to recall the events of a trip I made twenty years ago, the association Barjos—Abitibi is essential. To any of my present companions the words —let alone their connection—are nonsense; but, when I explain that I was wind-bound on an islet in Lake Abitibi for several days in company with an Indian named Barjos, both the words and the reason for their association are understood.

Now, when we speak of directed thinking, or when we study associations by ordinary introspective methods, we are dealing with associations that are either universally understood, comprehensible to some group, or immediately explicable by the subject. In all three cases, the background of experience, which rationalizes the associations, is available; and the thinking is directed, i.e. it is adaptive, because consciousness is oriented to a particular body of experience and is trying to solve some problem connected therewith. In our normal waking life, attention is so focussed on the immediate environment or on some body of experience that only the associations appropriate to the objects of attention come into consciousness. (If other associations occur we are not aware of them and should be justified in denying their existence, were it not for the presence of queer emotional reactions unaccounted for by any thought in consciousness.) There is, then, a correlation between maintenance of attention, adaptability of thinking and logicality of associations.

When attention is relaxed, however, undirected thinking begins to appear. More and more, apparently lawless associations occur —associations so illogical, so random, as to shock consciousness, if it be suddenly re-awakened, with a suggestion of mental disintegration. Such sequences Freud has termed "free associations". It cannot be too strongly emphasized that the ordinary introspectionist is quite ignorant of them and for an excellent reason. To examine them critically consciousness must be on the alert; when it is active, attention is focussed and the phenomenon does not take place.

Only those who have attempted the psycho-analytic method, on themselves or others, are aware of the difficulty of the experiment. It is, of course, impossible at the same instant to relax conscious control of one's thoughts and to scrutinize them critically. Alternation of these processes is, however, possible, although arduous. Those who have sincerely attempted to do this are well aware of how far from "free" the data actually secured for examination may be. The association may occur, for instance, as an image. The mere effort to focus attention on this, or to get it translated into words, is sufficient to cause it to melt away, leaving some idea or picture which the intelligent and honest subject knows is only a substitute. He then says: "I am thinking of such and such, but that's not what I thought of first. I just can't get a hold on the first thing". If his efforts are finally fruitful, the elusive idea or image is found to be represented more acceptably in the substitute.

There are two grounds for the inacceptability of the truly free association. One of these is that it is apt to express or imply some moral obliquity. This is the aspect which Freud has elaborated. Less attention has been paid to the other, although it has equal importance for the psychologist. The more intellectualized and conscious our living becomes, the more important to us does rationality seem. The self of which we are aware is rational and controls its thinking logically. This self, in the course of mental evolution, becomes precious and is treated as if it were life itself. What we call the instinct of self-preservation is, primitively, merely an impulse to avoid bodily injury. As the concept of self grows, it is the personality which must be protected. Finally, consciousness and its functions, which incorporate and express the highly civilized self, come under the protection of this basic instinct. The more self-conscious an individual is, the more does disintegration of this system—or any suggestion thereof—become a signal for a protective reaction, that is as instinctive as stepping out of the way of a motor car. This reaction naturally takes the form of a re-invigorated critique and elimination from consciousness of anything irrational. By definition an introspectionist is one with highly intellectual interests. For him a lapse of consciousness is, therefore, bound to entail greater discomfort than it would in a less self-conscious person. Since an inevitable feature of free associations is irrationality, it follows that the introspective psychologist is the last man in the world to study them in himself. To do so he must develop an interest in them so strong and so automatic as to be more powerful than the particular exhibition of the instinct of self-preservation we have been discussing. This is very hard to do: it is as difficult as it is for the would-be boxer to learn to direct his gaze away from the face of his opponent and not to shut his eyes as he wards off a blow towards his own face. If the psychologist begins with scepticism his initial experiments will prove to him that there are no such things as free associations.

Fortunately for our science, however, there are many forms of mental disease in which conscious critique is withdrawn in varying degrees and in which verbal productivity is still maintained. In such cases, the conditions of experiment are fulfilled, and we have the added advantage of dealing with truly objective material, for the consciousness scrutinizing the recorded associations has no connection with the mind that has produced them. A study of this material gives abundant confirmation to every claim that Freud has made as to the free associations procurable from normal, or merely psychoneurotic, subjects. It would, therefore, seem highly probable that the psycho-analyst's observations are sound. But it is expedient to argue from the more objective material, so I have tried to deduce the laws of free association from records made of verbal productions of the insane. It should be emphasized, however, that there is little that is original in this. Both the stimulus and clue were derived from Freudian theory. A large portion of my bulky book on Emotion is taken up with a presentation of the data on this subject and to it the interested reader is referred. Only generalizations derived from the data can be discussed here.

It has been argued above that the normality, or rationality, of associations is correlated with the maintenance of conscious functions, specifically with the adaptive orientation of attention. If this be so, the phenomena of free association ought to appear with greater frequency as the attempt, made by the patient to adapt himself to his environment and to his standards of thought and behaviour, grows weaker and weaker. In other words, the more insane he is, provided he remains verbally productive, the more apparently lawless his utterances should become. This is easily shewn to be the case, and a scale may be drawn up demonstrating the growing "freedom" of associations as adaptive attention wanes.

We may begin with the cases of *hypomania*, that is of a state of mild excitement that grades over insensibly into normal elation. These patients shew a heightened physical activity, a relatively unbridled emotionality (usually elation), and great talkativeness. Alcohol produces just this picture in many people. Superficial study of what they say seems to shew that they are simply drifting from one joke, from one boastful reminiscence, to another and that any chance environmental stimulus may distract their attention. If, however, one takes the trouble to make extensive records of their utterances, it is found that, in spite of their distractibility and rambling sequence, the range of topics is really surprisingly small. Certain memories, references to certain people and certain interests, are constantly recurring; most surprising of all, it is only *some* environmental stimuli which are repeatedly distracting them. This narrow range of topics we have called the trend of ideas, or, for short, simply "trend". The trend is something of highly individual and personal significance, and it is intruded on the auditor without consideration of politeness, nor, often enough, of intelligibility. It would seem, therefore, that what produces this trend is some inner interest, stronger, for the time being, than the force directing adaptive intelligence, and capable of selecting topics germane to itself. An intelligent patient once described these phenomena as follows: "On the whole I feel that when I am exhilarated, my mind occupies itself, for the most part, with its own affairs. And its inspiration and motives for action are self-creative and come from within. It is, as a rule, too busy, and in too much of a hurry, to stop and make minute, rational, and detailed account in passing of external objects. Its tendency is towards flightiness." As a matter of fact, the florid development, of such relatively maladaptive thinking is known to psychiatrists as "flight of ideas".

In these states adaptiveness is still sufficiently retained to ensure an approximately grammatical sentence structure, and the auditor can make a fair guess as to the nature of the interests and experiences in the background which have supplied the basis for the associations recorded. If too ignorant of the patient's life and interests to make this guess, an examiner can often get him to explain the connection. The background, then, is still of the normal order; all that has happened is that egocentric, rather than externalized, interests have begun to determine the direction of attention.

When we turn from these mild excitements to the severe ones, that are labelled as *mania*, the connections between successive verbal utterances are by no means so easily understood or discoverable. The background which rationalizes the associations is no longer universal, nor esoteric: it does not seem at first blush to be even personal in many instances, for after recovery the patient may be unable to explain the sequence. On the other hand, other links, irrational but obvious, appear. Comments on the environment may be uttered in an order that seems to follow the wandering attention of the patient. Or purely sound (*Klang*) associations may be prominent. When sound associations, distractibility and "nonsense", provide many of the links between consecutive elements in the stream of speech, we speak of "flight of ideas". Loss of adaptability is further evidenced by a progressive, syntactical degradation. Sentence structure tends to lapse in favour of disjointed phrases or even of grammatically ununited words. If this divagation from normality continues still further, the externalized expression of thoughts in spoken words may be abandoned, while at the same time these thoughts are presented more and more to the patient as images—or at least so a large amount of evidence would indicate. This whole process, including all its stages, I have termed "Distraction of Thought".[1]

Superficially viewed the process seems to be a negative one, with the exception of the factors of distractibility and sound

[1] *Psychology of Emotion*, chap. XXIII.

association which are obviously intruded. That is, rational bonds are loosed, as adaptability weakens, and what is left is *non*sense; the resulting associations are lawless. So it has seemed to the conventional psychiatrist, and elaborate physiologies of the brain have been invented to account for the insanity, for the chance connections that seem to be due to "crossed wires". The theory of chance is given a death-blow, however, by a simple, although time-consuming, experiment, which any psychiatrist can make. If a stenographic record be made of *everything* which a manic patient says at one interview, and a similar record be taken at a later date—after days, weeks, or months have elapsed, even in a subsequent attack years after—a comparison of the two will shew an astonishing proportion of the nonsensical associations to be repeated. Still more striking is the fact that identical comments may be made on the same environmental data after long intervals of time. If the laws governing these "chance" associations were only the mathematical ones of probability, repetitions would be the exception rather than the rule. The change from normal to abnormal associations is, then, not a result of the loss of a single factor—adaptability—some other factor has entered in. What this is appears when the repetitious elements are collated. Properly arranged and interpreted in the light of the patient's career, they make up a story: it is again the "trend". But it is now a slightly different story. Ask the hypomanic patient after recovery about his trend and he will admit it all. He may apologize for some of it as representing rather fantastic ambitions, but he recognizes them as his. On the other hand if the manic patient be similarly questioned he may deny a number of the ideas imputed to him. It is not merely the implications of his remarks that he denies; he will even claim that the record has been falsified, that he never said nor could have said the words imputed to him. Yet there they are, forming integral elements in a theme that rationalizes practically every word of what, at first sight, seemed a meaningless jumble. Are we to omit meaningful elements just because the subject has forgotten his mention of them? Or, are we to follow Freud's lead and regard such data as "unconscious" in origin? So long as the number of these tabooed ideas is relatively small we may, perhaps, avoid the rendering of a decision. But when we turn to many cases of *dementia praecox* and find such material bulking larger than the "normal", the dilemma must be faced.

In this disease there occurs a curious distortion of thinking, known as "scattered speech", which is psychologically correlated with the general disintegration that characterizes this chronic psychosis. In scattered speech sentence structure is, as a rule, preserved but the sequence is superficially senseless. It seems like a mere jumble of words and in its extreme form has been called a "word salad". An old and naïve theory was that some kind of cerebral disintegration caused association paths to be mixed up. The more modern view, based on many painstaking studies, is that the patient has given special meanings to a series of words: these personal, individual meanings alternate with those in current use, so that the same word may be used in quite different senses even in one sentence. It is the alternation of literal with metaphorical or symbolic meanings that causes the confusion. If the latter be discovered and expressed directly, an intelligible statement is disclosed. For instance a patient may say, "He kicked the door and she had a baby". If it be known that forcing a door in any way is a symbol for sexual intercourse, the sequence of ideas is no longer nonsensical.

A frequent mode of assimilating two words is their similarity in sound. This leads many a dementia praecox patient to the fabrication of atrocious puns, puns so far-fetched that their silliness seems sufficient proof of sound association alone accounting for the word conjunction. A deeper connection is frequently discoverable, however, a connection that is discerned only when the patient's individual meanings have been ferreted out, when a glossary of his peculiar "language" has been compiled. I once made an arduous study of the verbal productions of a dementia praecox patient, whose torrential flow of words was, at first blush, utterly incomprehensible.[1] By innumerable cross-references among the ideas associated, a key to his code was finally worked out. It was then seen that a large number of words were symbolizing a relatively small group of concepts and that the latter gave expression to a banal delusional story. Excruciating puns provided

---

[1] Three examples may make this plain: "I don't doubt the ocean pays freight. A man who watches those steamers and brings them into his home every day, he is an educated man". "Music is simply a sound, but to be produced it must be agitated. Sufficient agitation produces such sound. The father pays for the daughter and the mother for the daughter. Quintrillions of words falling into spittoons all over the world. I don't care for that man." "A locomotive is an infant industry. When you knock the first piece of iron, that is a locomotive as good as made, that is a directory."

a facile mechanism for bringing two words together, but a deeper connection was always apparent when the code had been discovered. For example he once remarked: "What is gambling? Senno Gambia, the richest country in God's earth; it's down in Africa. That is the derivation of the word Senno Gambia." When it is known that *gambling* and *Africa* both stood for homosexuality and that *words* frequently meant spermatozoa, the sentences are not so nonsensical. The same patient spoke indifferently in French and English. Often his puns were bilingual: "Garibaldi is a French word—look, look, he is building [re*gar*der, *build*]. Heart disease says, gluck, gluck, gluck and the eye says look, look, look. The word of the heart or the word of the eye." This passage is more difficult, because the meaning of "building" was never determined with finality. "Garibaldi," however, was one of a number of people who represented his father, a Frenchman who had died of apoplexy, a disease, according to the patient's delusion, induced by excessive sexuality. If we assume that "building" means sexual activity (which is not inherently improbable, for practically every word he uttered referred either directly or symbolically to something sexual), then a meaning can be given to the sequence. It would be: Look at my French father's sexuality; it leads to a circulatory disease. Quite possibly the "eye" stands for head or brain, but that too remains a speculation, for my decoding of an unlimited amount of material had to stop at some point.

The principle followed in making such an analysis as this is exactly that of one who tries to find the meaning of slang terms without direct enquiry. Badly "scattered" patients will not co-operate, so that all that can be done is to learn the various settings in which a given word is used with apparent irrelevance. The statement "John Smith is a nut" means something quite different in America from what it does in England, but the context soon betrays the two meanings to a student of slang. Of course, with slang one can make direct enquiry, but, if the question be put to a gamin in the slums, the reply may only be more slang, so the parallel holds. Confirmation of the method is secured from the introspection of milder, and intelligent, dementia praecox patients, who will sometimes give exquisitely accurate accounts of double meanings of symbolic words and objects.[1]

[1] See, for instance, *Psychology of Emotion*, p. 422.

The assumption made either by the student of slang or the student of dementia praecox is that there exists, or has existed, some field of experience which rationalizes the apparently irrelevant conjunction of words. The slang or the symbol has grown up as a metaphor or by association through coincidence in time or place. This experience I have referred to above as the "background". If the background be known, the association is no longer meaningless. While writing this chapter, I have come across an excellent example from the pen of an eminent psychologist. He is speaking of the importance of external circumstance in the determination of a scale of values and the difficulty of reducing these to any measurable units. He goes on: "In the absence of measures one depends on opinion, and those competent to weigh their experiences will not have had average ones. The elephant is very like a rope." The last statement, taking it at its face value, was as incomprehensible to me as any bit of scattered speech. Knowing the author personally, however, no suspicion of dementia praecox crossed my mind. I was familiar with his penchant for cryptic expression and so assumed at once that the background was not personal but esoteric. A fable seemed the most likely basis, but I could not bring an appropriate one to mind. Before long, I naturally was able to get the explanation from a friend. It was the tale of several blind men who examined different parts of an elephant and so gave widely different accounts of the structure of the animal: the one who seized his tail avowed that the elephant was very like a rope. On hearing the fable recited, it was familiar to me, but for lack of instantaneous memory thereof a reference to it had been meaningless.

It cannot be too strongly emphasized that I have chosen to use pathological material here merely on account of its simplicity and objective character. Precisely the same principles are exemplified in "free associations" as elicited during psycho-analysis. Indeed it is not necessary to go so far afield. If anyone takes the pains— it is truly difficult—to follow his mental processes as he is falling asleep he will discover that, with the relaxation of externalized interest, associations become less logical, connected by more and more purely personal links and tend to assume an imaginal form. This process eventually gives rise to dreaming, in which the thinking is entirely of the irrational order that I have been describing.[1]

---

[1] *Psychology of Emotion*, chap. XLIX.

The most important feature of "undirected" thinking remains to be discussed. I have mentioned that the verbal productions of the manic patient shew a strikingly high proportion of repetitions. When these are examined and collated they make up the "trend". If this were an elaborate tale it would have little significance for our present purpose. But the reverse is true: it is a simple theme whose variations are superficial and trivial. Items of past and present experience, that seem to reflect a wide range of circumstance or interest, do, it is true, form the apparent fabric of the patients' display; but when its composition is scrutinized a fundamental design is seen to have brought the diverse elements together. And this design is a small series of simple, unconscious strivings and aversions that are interrelated. Once the trend is reconstructed, many of the patient's characteristics while normal are explained at the same time that his insane fantasies and preoccupations are rationalized. Any kind of object, idea, or activity, that can serve as a symbol for the unconscious motivations, is woven into the tapestry. In normal life these symbols are selected and arranged so as to form a logical sequence that conceals the underlying principle of choice. But in the psychosis, associations having become "free" as reason departs, the hidden agency is disclosed. The plot being revealed, the many actors, each of whom has seemed to have his own personality, are seen to be but puppets. An analogy from everyday life is pertinent. We are all familiar with the political or economic theorist who can find a text for the ventilation of his pet remedy in the most diverse and apparently unrelated events. So does the unconscious *idée fixe* utilize a large variety of elements in its construction of characteristics or symptoms.

The trend, then, can be boiled down to quite a simple story. But this is not all. In a large series of cases it is found that the same themes are recurring with a wearying iteration, so that it is possible to establish a greatest common measure, as it were, among the unconscious factors detected by this kind of analysis. Moreover, it is often surprising to discover how little is left over when this greatest common measure is subtracted from the trend in any individual case. We are thus enabled to arrive at a most important generalization. A dynamic agency, so independent of varying circumstance as to reappear in the mental life of rich and poor, bond and free, must have something instinctive in it. And, indeed, it is not difficult to identify and catalogue the instincts—or instinct groups—that are responsible for the trends of our patients. This, however, is not our present task, which is merely to shew the derivation of the theory which states that there are unconscious and instinctive agencies underlying our conscious mental life. These agencies I shall call *patterns*. With our multiform capacities of adaptation to a constantly changing environment and with our subjective experience of volition, it takes a peculiarly honest and penetrating introspection to detect the presence in our mental life of a foundation of set modes of reaction. But, when both psychopathology and genetic psychology have demonstrated its probability, introspection can go a long way towards confirming the theory.

It may be well to summarize the argument of this chapter. When we study the nature of the connections uniting consecutive elements in trains of thought, the "background" or experiential basis for the associations is seen to shift. As we leave directed thinking and penetrate further and further into the apparently lawless wanderings of the mind, we discover that these are not controlled by consciousness and not by efforts of adaptation to the environment, but are oriented by inner forces. Instead of the associations springing from the universally recognized meanings of the entities occurring in the flux, we find a background that is first esoteric, then individual and finally unconscious. Parallelling this change in derivation of meaning, the form of the thoughts is altered with a gradual substitution of images for abstract thoughts until finally the flux is purely imaginal. The sequence of these images is not a matter of chance but is determined by patterns, i.e. agencies of an instinctive order that control the direction of a series of mental reactions.

This is thinking in its most primitive human form. That it occurs in all of us during emergencies, when we behave "instinctively", would be admitted by anyone. Of recent years, however, the researches of psychopathologists have led to the theory being propounded that this kind of mental process can exist outside of conscious awareness, parallelling the thinking revealed to introspection and serving as a foundation for the latter. We are indebted as much to the observations of the hypnotists—particularly to Morton Prince—as we are to the Freudians for the data from which this hypothesis is deduced. If this view be sound, we

ought to be able to reconstruct the mental life of man as a combination and interaction of pattern and conscious thinking. Before
attempting to do so, it will be advisable to examine the structure
of simple patterns and to arrive at some understanding of what
we mean by consciousness.

CHAPTER IV

THE CONSTRUCTION OF PRIMITIVE
MENTAL PATTERNS

THE statement that our mental life is based on a series of reactions the direction of which is controlled by patterns is one with which few behaviourists would be likely to quarrel. When to this is added the claim that the patterns are composed of connected imaginal processes, a number of behaviourists would agree, provided this "image" were defined as an internal reaction of the organism. They would, of course, protest that "image" was a bad term because it implied something not directly reducible to physiological (i.e. physical and chemical) concepts. All of them would deny the value of ever trying to discuss the interaction of patterns with consciousness, for to them consciousness is not a psychological phenomenon but at best a premature hypothesis. The scheme I am trying to elaborate has, however, some affiliations with behaviourism. It may be well, therefore, to see how far the present scheme is behaviouristic and at what point, or points, a difference appears.

The behaviourist bases his system on the discoveries of biologists of "chain reflexes" and on the phenomena studied by physiologists of "conditioned reflexes". "Patterns" of behaviour are built up, he says, by conditioning responses to external stimuli into chains. Let us begin with an examination of chain reflexes.

This term was first used by Exner and popularized by Jacques Loeb. Essentially the notion is of an extended activity being analysable into elements; each of the latter is a separate reaction elicited by a new stimulus. The orderly sequence results from the fact that the first movement produces such a change as to bring the stimulus for the next reaction into operation, the second induces the third stimulus, and so on. A simple example is that of swallowing. It looks like a unitary sequence, but experiment has shewn that the gullet really works in segments. Food forced in at the top sets up a stimulus for contraction of the ring of muscle just above the bolus. The food is thus forced lower, and again the same reaction takes place. The end result is a steadily progressive wave of contraction always occurring just behind the food. A more complicated example of this principle has been demonstrated by Benedict Friedlaender.[1] The crawling movements of the earthworm consist of alternate lengthening and shortening of the whole body; microscopic bristles on its "belly" being pointed backwards, the head end is fixed when the shortening occurs so that the tail moves forward, while the tail being held by the bristles, when lengthening occurs, the head end slides forward. There are two series of muscles, a set of rings that are obviously segmental and longitudinal bands that are anatomically continuous. It would seem as if the earthworm's "brain" directed the contraction of these longitudinal muscles whose contraction shortens the body as a whole. But Friedlaender found that if the nerves were cut, or even if the whole animal were cut in two and tied together with strings, appropriate alternating contractions in both sets of muscles occur in the tail half. Apparently, movement of the front half causes a stretching of the skin in the latter half, and this serves as the stimulus for the contraction of the local longitudinal muscles. It is, therefore, assumed that the movement as a whole is compounded of a series of segmental contractions, even if they are synchronized. We shall have to refer later to the rôle of the nervous system in such co-ordinations as this, which can be accomplished without it.

A variety of senses may be employed in receiving the series of stimuli in a chain reflex. For instance sight, tactile and muscle sense enter into the so-called dart reflex of the frog, the movements which result in an insect being caught and swallowed. Sight of an insect is the stimulus for darting out the tongue at it. The touch of the foreign body on the tongue produces a closure of the mouth, while this last leads to swallowing.

Loeb takes as his simplest elements tropisms. These are responses of living matter to simple physical or chemical stimuli such as light (heliotropism), gravity (geotropism), or heat (thermotropism). In every case there is a movement towards the stimulus on the part of the organ or organism, or away from it if the tropism be a negative one. Tropisms are such primitive responses that

[1] Quoted by Loeb in *Comparative Physiology of the Brain and Comparative Psychology.*

they may be independent of any nervous tissue whatever; they are, indeed, characteristic of plants. Geotropism and heliotropism cause roots to strike into the earth and leaves to turn to the light. Loeb has gone so far as to attempt to account for instincts as mere chains of tropisms. It may be worth while to quote one of his examples.

"We find another instance of a preservative instinct in the young caterpillars of many butterflies. The larvae of *Porthesia chrysorrhoea* creep out of the eggs in the autumn and winter in colonies in a nest on trees or shrubs. The warm spring sun drives them out of the nest and they crawl up on the branches of the tree or shrub to the tip, where they find their first food. After having eaten the tips, they crawl about until they find new buds or leaves, which in the meantime have come out in great numbers. It is evident that the instinct of the caterpillars to crawl upwards, so soon as they awake from the winter's sleep, saves their lives. Were they not guided by such an instinct, those that crawl downwards would die of starvation....

"I have found that the young caterpillars of *Porthesia* are oriented by the light. Until they have taken food they are positively heliotropic. This positive heliotropism leads them to the tips of the branches where they find their food. During the winter they are stiff and do not move. The higher temperature of the spring brings about chemical changes in their bodies and these chemical processes cause them to move. But the direction of their movements is determined by the light. Out-of-doors, where the diffused light strikes the animal on all sides, every ray of light can be resolved into a horizontal and a vertical component, the horizontal components destroy each other, and only the effect of the vertical components remains. Hence the animals are forced, as a result of their positive heliotropism, to crawl upwards until they reach the tip of a branch. They are held there by the light. The chemical stimuli which are transmitted to the animal by the young buds produce the eating movements. In this instinct, which is necessary for the preservation of life, we have another instance of simple positive heliotropism....

"We have seen, however, that these same caterpillars leave the tips of the branches as soon as they have eaten and crawl downward. Why does the light not hold them on the highest point permanently? My experiments showed that these caterpillars are only positively heliotropic as long as they remain unfed; after having eaten they lose their positive heliotropism. This is not the only instance of this kind, for I have found a series of facts which show that chemical changes influence the irritability of the animal toward light...."

Similar observations on some sea worms led Loeb to account for their migrations on the basis of changing tropisms. When cold they are positively phototropic and so swim upwards in the water till they reach a warmer zone. When hot they become negatively phototropic and so descend. The nett result is that they migrate to levels of suitable temperature. He gives many such examples of adaptive behaviour that seem purposeful but on analysis turn out to be a series of responses to a changing set of stimuli, each change being effected by the previous reaction of the organism. It is often surprising to find how dependent an animal is on an appropriate external stimulus for the performance of an act that seems to be an integral part of a unified programme. For instance, a dog seeing food on the other side of a railing will make unhesitatingly a wide detour to get it. But, if the food be near enough to smell, he may try unavailingly and long to get at it directly.[1] The explanation is: pursuit of food is a reaction initiated by sight, whereas smell precipitates simply the act of seizing it. Again, it is stated that male rabbits whose olfactory nerves have been cut are unable to breed. Apparently the long train of behaviour constituting copulation must be initiated by the primary recognition of the doe in heat, which is accomplished by smell, or it will not occur at all.

Those who believe in the chain reflex theory would account for the behaviour of a cat catching a mouse somewhat as follows. Visceral disturbances, which we label as hunger, set up a reaction of mere restlessness; the animal wanders about. A small grey object is seen, which is the stimulus for a stalking progression towards the small grey object. When sufficient detail is perceived, or the mouse is actually smelt, a springing movement is liberated. Actual contact of the paws with the body of the prey causes the claws to be extruded, then the jaws to descend, and so forth. It may, perhaps, be convenient to represent this in a formula. If a, b, c, d, etc., are the stimuli, and α, β, γ, etc., are the motor responses, then the formula would be:

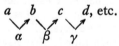

If this formula told the whole truth about animal behaviour, the cat, for example, would be entirely at the mercy of the environment. It would stalk the ball of grey wool on the floor when it was hungry; but we know that it does not. Sherrington says, in discussing the chain instinct theory, that there really is a selection

[1] Koehler, *Mentality of Apes*, p. 13.

of stimuli: "the threshold of each succeeding reflex is lowered by the excitation just preceding its own". The hungry cat has a lowered threshold for perception of its prey so that it responds selectively to the mouse or bird. This lowered threshold marks the beginning of a pattern—liminal images of the successive stimuli have appeared, to use my nomenclature—and this gives a general direction to the train of behaviour that otherwise would be as haphazard as the accidents of the environment could make it. When not all, but only some, stimuli are reacted to what appears to the human observer like purpose appears.

But there is still another objection to the formula. As integration of the pattern improves, still further independence of the environment is achieved; as I would say, some liminal images become image functions. In cases where the behaviour is fully adaptive, the reaction to something that is not there may not be obvious. But, where the impetus of the patterned behaviour causes the animal to react to a stimulus *before* it has physically appeared, the resultant premature act is maladaptive and, therefore, obvious. As an example we may take the phenomena reported by A. H. H. Fraser[1] in the lambing sheep. According to him, the following is the normal sequence of behaviour. As labour becomes imminent the sheep leaves the flock, seeking some isolated spot. There it makes a bed in which parturition takes place. When the lamb is born, the mother licks it and suckles it. Finally, both mother and off-spring return to the flock. Fraser has worked out the specific stimuli for each of these steps. From the shepherd's standpoint an embarrassing break in the chain often occurs and to this we may give special attention. The stimulus for the "maternal instinct" (i.e. attachment to the offspring) seems to be licking the lamb. This, of course, ought only to happen when the lamb is born. Unfortunately, however, when the membranes have come into the birth canal, the threshold for the maternal reaction is so low that the sheep may leave its bed and pursue a lamb detected by sight or sound at a considerable distance. This lamb is "adopted" and once it is licked the sheep will not leave it. Since licking inhibits labour pains, this practice of "lamb theft" may lead to the death of the unborn lamb. It is interesting that it occurs chiefly in old ewes.

[1] "Chain Instincts in Lambing Sheep," *Brit. Jour. Psychol.* vol. XVI, part 4, 1926.

Putting this in anthropomorphic terms, we should say that the ewe behaves as if she thought her lamb were already born and that she ought to find it—she may be induced at this stage to follow a bundle of white rags! In the chain instinct terminology it might be said that one step in the series of reactions was suppressed. If the anthropomorphic formulation implies quite unjustifiable assumptions, the chain instinct account errs in the opposite way, for it fails to account for a response to a stimulus that is distant, faint and incomparably less potent physiologically than the birth pains. It is not adequate to say that the stage of actual parturition is suppressed for the ewe behaves *as if it had taken place*. My nomenclature, I imagine, will get around both these difficulties. I should say that the total pattern "parturition-mothering" is becoming integrated into more of a single unit, that is, it is growing more or less independent of the physical presence of some stimuli originally necessary for the production of the several reactions now integrated together. When this integration has been achieved, the behaviour is as if the materially absent stimulus were there, and the apparent operation of this absent stimulus I call an image function. It cannot be too strongly emphasized that the term "image function" implies absolutely nothing as to the organism's subjective state. It is merely a label to cover a kind of reaction that is objectively observed. Whether this label is useful or pernicious remains to be seen, but there can be no doubt as to the existence of the phenomenon which it denotes.

This brings us to a preliminary discussion of the experimental production of image functions, that is to say of "conditioned reflexes". For our present purposes we need consider only a single, but fundamental, experiment, that has been repeated so many times as to leave no doubt whatever as to the facts. If a dog be presented with some food a flow of saliva will take place. This is an inborn, or "unconditioned", reflex. If this procedure be repeated a sufficient number of times, and, if on each occasion a whistle is blown just before the food is produced, the dog will eventually salivate when the whistle is blown, although no food whatever is offered. This is now a "conditioned reflex"; the whistle is the "conditioned stimulus" and the food the "unconditioned stimulus". The auditory stimulus has somehow become associated with the reaction of salivation so that it produces the latter. The experiment has been performed with a great variety of inborn reflexes and of conditioned stimuli in a number of animals and children. The results are sufficiently constant to justify this general formula: A previously irrelevant stimulus may produce a given reflex action when that stimulus has been presented in association with the stimulus appropriate for the reaction in question. The number of repetitions required varies with the nature of the reactions and with the "intelligence" of the animal. In man one experience of the associated stimuli may often be sufficient, and this is seen in some dogs as well, particularly when the reaction has a strong "emotional" colouring. I may cite one observation of my own in substantiation of this statement. I was once starting out for a walk with my dog—a Great Dane aged three and a quarter years—and was passing through a yard of the stables where he lived. A cat with two kittens appeared and the dog started to attack them. I called out a condemnatory word and he cringed. A few days later, in precisely the same place, the cat again appeared. Again the dog lunged towards it, but, without a sign from me (so far as I was aware), checked his assault almost in mid-air, cringed, and came fawning towards me.

This reaction differs from the laboratory results only in its surprising, almost dramatic, quality. To the old-fashioned, sentimental dog-lover the explanation is easy: the dog remembered in time that he was doing wrong and turned to apologize to me. Unfortunately for this interpretation, during the years of observation of this dog, very few examples of behaviour were displayed which seemed capable of explanation only on a basis of conscious thinking such as human beings are subjectively aware of. It seemed rather that his intelligence consisted merely—or almost entirely—of a facility in the formation of conditioned responses, which, once formed, were repeated blindly, inevitably, even against his "interests". The anthropomorphic formula seems, therefore, to be unscientific. The various Russians, chiefly Pavlov and his pupils, who have done such magnificent work in this field, give physiological and mechanistic explanations of these conditioned reflexes. Later[1] we shall have to examine these (and may find them—mechanistically—untenable), but for the present our terminology ought to be psychological. The animals react as if a stimulus experienced in the past were again in operation. For this we have coined the term "image function". We should, therefore,

---

[1] In a subsequent book.

say that when my dog cringed there was in operation an image function of my voice—or, more vaguely and so more accurately, of my threat.

From this point we can go on to examine the problem of how a series of responses to external stimuli—the chain reflex—can gain independence of the environment while it becomes integrated into a unitary whole. When an animal reacts to two stimuli in succession, there are two ways in which conditioning may take place. The first is exemplified in the conditioning of a sound stimulus with salivation. The note of the whistle produces a reaction of orientation—pricking-up of the ears, etc. While this orientation is in progress, food is shewn and salivation commences. Unless the interval between the two is very long, salivation occurs in response to a stimulus complex that includes both sound and the sight of food. As this is repeated oftener and oftener, the orientation response, which is a fairly inconspicuous one even at the outset, merges over more and more into the salivation. Finally, the orientation in response to this particular sound becomes an orientation to food alone, that is, *this particular orientation is salivation.* The sight of food has become an image function.

This accounts for one environmental stimulus being dropped; but it is a case where one reaction merges naturally over into another. Orientation is a diffuse response that is largely a heightened excitability favouring any kind of a sequential reaction. Another explanation is required for the conditioning together of reactions that are different in kind, which is what must occur if a chain of responses are to be unified into an integrated whole. What link can there be apart from the intertwining of the reactions themselves?

For this second explanation a factor must be reckoned with of which we have so far taken no account. When a muscle contracts, or is passively stretched, sensory nerve endings in the muscles, tendons and joints are stimulated. These sensory nerves belong to the general proprioceptive system. (That is, sensory nerves transmitting the effects of changes initiated within the body.) If, when one reaction is in progress, a stimulus tending to produce a response of another kind is thrown in, the total sensory situation includes not merely the new environmental stimulus but also the proprioceptive stimuli set up by the first reaction. With sufficient repetition of the sequence these stimuli from internal and external sources may be conditioned together. For instance, in a reciprocal movement mere stretching of some muscles to a certain point will become an adequate stimulus for contraction of the opposing set of muscles. The walking reflex is thus composed as has been amply demonstrated in the physiological laboratory. That proprioceptive stimuli can function as conditioning stimuli has been fully demonstrated by experiment in the laboratories of Pavlov and Beritoff. By this means, reflexes involving muscular movements of quite different kinds can be integrated together with the elimination of the environmental stimulus for the second reaction, i.e. its appearance only as an image function. The extent to which a material agency may become unnecessary for the production of its specific physiological effect was shewn in the course of Krylov's experiments with morphine in dogs.[1] After they had become accustomed to injections of morphine, the mere sight of a hypodermic syringe would produce nausea with salivation, followed by vomiting and sleep, these symptoms being originally the effect of morphine after it had been absorbed and was circulating in the blood. This is, of course, analogous to the sea-sickness that overtakes some unfortunate human subjects on walking up the gang-plank.

So far we have considered the types of experiment which demonstrate that environmental stimuli can become image functions. The result of this process is to make possible the repetition of a series of reactions, *provided* each one of these actions actually occurs or is developed to a point sufficient for the production of proprioceptive stimuli. This, however, is not a completely integrated pattern, for each reaction of the series is still made in response to an actual stimulus. (It must be borne in mind that, from the standpoint of the functioning of the central nervous system, the body as a whole is the environment. Every stimulus, no matter whether it originates within or without the body, affects the central nervous system as a result of a bodily disturbance.) In other words, we are still dealing with a chain of reflexes that is not less a chain because the serial stimuli are not obvious to the observer. A question of fundamental importance now arises: Can integration proceed further; specifically, can the proprioceptive stimulus become an image function? If it cannot, the principle

[1] As reported by Pavlov, *Conditioned Reflexes*, translated by G. V. Anrep, Oxford Univ. Press, 1927, p. 35.

of parsimony would justify us in putting our psychology on a basis of mechanistic physiology. If it can, behaviourism is only a useful method of studying animal behaviour and not a defensible system of psychology. The issue can be narrowed down to this one point.

Behaviourism began as a revolt—and a justifiable one—against the anthropomorphism of the earlier introspective psychology which ascribed conscious thinking to the lower animals. Originally behaviourism was a method of approach to the study of animal behaviour; it set out to discover how much animal reactions could be formulated in terms of fixed responses to set stimuli. That is, its method was to be purely objective. Beginning with the chain reflex hypothesis, amended and enlarged by uniting it with the principles of conditioned reflexes, the behaviourists arrived at the conclusion that all animal behaviour could be accounted for on the basis of inborn or acquired patterns of response to given stimuli. New responses, new adaptations, were to be regarded not as the product of "reasoning" but as new conditioned reflexes: intelligence was merely a facility in the establishment of new responses. (My argument so far in this chapter has been, essentially, the behaviouristic one, except for the use of the term image function which has implications the behaviourist would not sanction.) Turning to babies and small children, both observation of spontaneous and experimental reactions seemed to shew only the same principles at work. Finally, it was found that much of the so-called reasoned behaviour of adult man could be adequately described in terms that took no account of consciousness. A safe, conservative conclusion from all this would be that patterns of behaviour, such as we have been describing, constitute the basic mental structure common to all the higher animals including man. Unfortunately many behaviourists have, in their enthusiasm, tried to elevate this generalization into a psychological theory covering all mental reactions, even those of the most intelligent man. We need not tarry to criticize such extravagant claims.[1] But even those who

---

[1] "We need nothing to explain behaviour but the ordinary laws of physics and chemistry." "The behaviourist cannot find consciousness in the test-tube of his science." Is that the place to look for it? Yet this same writer (John B. Watson) cannot describe phenomena of human psychology without using not merely the language of introspection but also its concepts. For instance, he writes: "Both [parents] are trying to recreate the child in their own image". A circumlocution might translate this volition into terms of conditioned responses, but how about the image and a composite one at that?

are too wise to make such boasts would seem to harbour a hope that physics and chemistry may one day be able to justify the hypothesis: else why do they insist on the inutility of dealing with subjective material? Specifically they dispute the expedience of using either the term image or, indeed, the concept of imaginal processes in general.

An excellent example of their arguments is to be found in the classical paper of Walter S. Hunter on "The Delayed Reaction in Animals and Children".[1] I single it out for criticism because it is the work of a skilled experimenter, who stands justifiably high in the estimate of psychologists, and it was undertaken in an effort to gather data on our very problem. Moreover the essentials of his experimental findings have not been called in question since they were published in 1913.

Hunter used twenty-two rats, two dogs, four raccoons, four children from six to eight years of age and one girl of two and a half years. With the animals the reaction was first conditioned of going through one of three holes to get food, there being a light over the hole where the food was. The animals were held in a kind of cage equidistant from all three holes and learned to go to whichever hole was indicated by the light, so soon as released. Then the light was turned off at increasing intervals of time before the animals could reach the hole; later, the light was turned off before the animal was released at all. Analogous apparatus and method was used with the children. All the experiments were obviously well controlled, so that when the delay was of any length the only possible cues used by the animals in going to the correct hole were internal. Rats were successful in going to the right hole with delays up to ten seconds; the dogs succeeded up to five minutes; the raccoons up to twenty-five seconds; the older children up to twenty-five minutes, but the little girl of two and a half only up to fifty seconds. It was observed that the rats and dogs succeeded only if they maintained their bodily orientation towards the right hole during the period of delay. (This orientation might amount to no more than a fixed direction of the head.) Raccoons used such orientation with obvious frequency, but both they and the children could be markedly distracted from it and still give a high proportion of correct responses.

"...as soon as a stage is reached where the determining stimuli

---

[1] *Behavior Monographs*, vol. II, no. 1.

are absent at the moment of reaction, then it is necessary, I assume, if the reactions are to succeed, that the subject develope substitutes which shall take the place of those stimuli as carriers of the needed meanings. In other words, the substitutes must *fulfil the function* of the previous stimuli in arousing the three appropriate movements....In view of the fact that delayed reactions did succeed under the present conditions, there can be no question as to the *existence* of the substitutes." He grants the existence of images in the case of the children whose introspective testimony, spontaneously offered, declared it. There remains the problem of the nature of substitutive stimulus in the raccoons.

"Some unknown intra-organic cue not observable by the experimenter" must be used. "The data...conclusively prove that the maintenance of orientation during the delay was an essential condition for correct response with the rats and dogs, and that such motor attitudes exerted a strong influence upon the behaviour of the raccoons....These orientation attitudes, like any sensory process, may be a stimulus to definite movements." Hunter assumes that the reactions in the total chain were conditioned in the following order historically: food taking and entering the hole, then entering the hole marked by a light, then movements towards the lighted hole, then orientation for this movement and finally release with the orientation. After delay the release stimulates the orientation reaction which provides the necessary cue. The correct choice out of three possible orientation reactions he assigns to the fact that the correct one was the one most recently stimulated, i.e. by the light.

If the proprioceptive stimuli aroused by the muscle tensions in orientation recur after the muscles in question are engaged in quite other responses, these proprioceptive stimuli must be of an imaginal nature in their revival. Hunter argues that choice is determined by some representation of the light, which might be a "sensation arising from the reagent's body—kinaesthetic, e.g.—that stands for a certain reaction...". The argument which justifies him in speaking of this internal agency as a sensation rather than as something imaginal is a curious one.

The light, he says, is somehow represented. If it be represented by an internal sensation (kinaesthetic), it will not be necessary to consider it an image. In human introspection we have knowledge of a number, for instance, being remembered by saying it aloud and then consigning it to "the preservative tendencies". The recall of this motor (speech) reaction is not experienced as an image, but has been called a "conscious attitude" in the language of introspective psychology. Hunter thinks it might just as well be called "sensory thought", i.e. sensations plus meaning. He does not enter into any analysis of the meaning component to shew that it can be reduced to simple stimulus and response elements, but merely elaborates the "sensory" component. "Raccoons and young children are capable of reactions that seem explicable only on the assumption of the functional efficiency of a representative factor. If sensations *can* function in this manner, the law of parsimony forbids the assumption of images." He leaves quite untouched the question of what is supplying the actual stimulus that constitutes the "sensation". It seems to me that "sensory thought" is precisely my "image function".

He places the stage of sensory thought genetically before that of images. The latter are recognizable by introspection alone. "On the basis of human *introspection*, there is another grade or kind of learning, viz., the stage of functional efficiency of images or centrally aroused conscious processes. Why there should be both sensory and imaginal thought in human experience is very difficult to say. The most obvious suggestion would be that imaginal thought, since it is genetically later, could accomplish tasks which sensory thought could not. I shall hazard no guesses as to what such tasks might be."

This is an honest admission of the limitation of the field of behaviourism. But should its limitation not be still narrower? If stimulus and response formulae are everywhere to be employed therein, should not its theories compass only those phenomena where "representation" does not enter in? For Hunter has eliminated the word "image" only by verbal juggling (and an argument drawn from subjective human criteria), but he has not succeeded in eliminating the concept of imaginal processes even in animal behaviour.

It therefore seems to me that we are justified in accepting Hunter's experiments on delayed reactions as proof that proprioceptive stimuli can be reproduced as image functions. If this be so, we can take another, and an important, step in our theoretical reconstruction of patterns. We have already found experimental proof that a chain of responses may be continued in the material absence of the environmental stimuli that originally occasioned the several responses: we call this the operation of image functions of the materially absent stimuli. We have further seen that proprioceptive stimuli arising from one reaction may become the conditioned stimuli for the next in the chain. If, now, these proprioceptives can also have an imaginal reproduction, an imaginal reaction may become the effective stimulus for the next. If this, in turn, be imaginally reproduced, an increasing portion of the total pattern may exist only as image functions of both external stimuli and of the reactions to them. The pattern then becomes —after sufficient integration—a flux of image functions, the existence of which is deduced from the fact that a given objective stimulus leads, in overt action, not to its own proper response, but to a reaction belonging to a later stage in the total chain. The whole series of actual responses no longer needs to be rehearsed in actual movement. If we now assume that conscious awareness, such as man enjoys, be directed to these inner events, then introspection will discover a train of images.

The fundamental process involved in the formation of patterns is conditioning. In the lower forms of life, many repetitions are necessary for the establishment of even one image function; this means that only such patterns will be formed as represent the integrated responses to stimuli which the environment has furnished in proper sequence innumerable times. Such an organism is, then, peculiarly dependent on its environment. (We shall shortly be examining appetites and then learn how certain stimuli are sought, thus limiting the completeness of the dependence.) In the higher forms conditioning occurs with greater and greater facility. This means that, on the theory of probability, a constantly larger number of stimuli, as conditioning becomes more facile, will be encountered sufficiently often in conjunction to have their responses integrated. Such creatures will, therefore, possess much more complicated patterns than their phylogenetically more primitive forebears. In man the number of experiences necessary for conditioning is extremely small, in fact one experience may suffice to associate a considerable number of elements. This being so, it is easy to see how man may build up patterns of incredible complication—as, indeed, he does.

No matter how complicated they may be, however, such patterns as we have so far derived, remain the guiding agencies for set, generic modes of behaviour. They are discriminative only in the sense that they may exist in large numbers as modes of reaction to a large number of slightly varying situations. But, by themselves they cannot produce new behaviour adaptive to a new situation. (A man with nothing but these patterns would be as badly off as that equipment leaves him which is furnished in the formulae of the behaviourists.) This is equivalent to saying that patterns are instinctive in character. If, as has been remarked above, a series of image functions be revealed to introspection, they would appear as a flux of images. Now we have seen in the last chapter that a study of free associations in both health and disease indicated as a probable basis for our mental life imaginal processes directed in their sequence by instinctive trends. In this chapter exactly such processes have been derived genetically. But it must be borne in mind that, though these patterns may serve as an explanation of most of the behaviour of animals, they can only be regarded as constituting the *foundations* of human mental life. Such patterns, taken alone, are quite inadequate to explain the whole problem of human behaviour.

CHAPTER V

THE PRIMARY FUNCTION
OF CONSCIOUSNESS

THE images, or image functions, considered in the previous chapter function adaptively as links in a chain, i.e. as elements in a pattern. The imaginal process which leads directly to its appropriate response, effected in actual, overt behaviour, is maladaptive. It is identical—objectively—with the phenomenon of hallucination in the insane, because it is a reaction to something that is not there. If, however, it leads to the excitation of more image functions, to the activation of a pattern, the resultant behaviour may bring the animal eventually into the presence of the real, rather than the imaginal, stimulus. Two examples may make this contrast clear. When a dog salivates on hearing a whistle blown, he acts as if he had just taken food, which is surely a maladaptive performance. On the other hand, if a whistle be blown and he comes running to be fed, that action is adaptive, or at least it well may be. In this latter instance, it is not necessary to assume that he consciously images the acquisition of food, but merely that a repetition of stimuli and their responses has produced an integration of the responses into a pattern that may be adaptive. We may conclude, therefore, that imaginal processes are adaptive only in so far as they are integrated to other image functions, but that they are definitely maladaptive when occurring in isolation. Yet our introspection teaches us that we can discern images as separable units, as existing apart from the flux in which they may appear. Moreover our experience tells us that such isolated images may be highly useful to us. Furthermore we know that they are useful when we are aware of them but recognize them to be images and not perceptions of something in the environment. In other words, the utilization of images is bound up with consciousness.

What is consciousness? It may as well be admitted, at the outset, that no definition can be given of it which will satisfy everybody, for the simple reason that few people—even psychologists—use the term consistently. A word whose use is fluid will not be defined satisfactorily when it is given a restricted meaning, for that impoverishes the loose thinker.

The *Concise Oxford Dictionary* defines "consciousness" as: "State of being conscious; totality of a person's thoughts and feelings, or of a class of these, as *moral consciousness*; perception (*of, that*)". "Conscious" in turn is defined as: "Aware, knowing, (*of* fact, *of* external circumstances, *that*, or absolute); with mental faculties awake; (of things) felt, sensible; equals SELF-CONSCIOUS." Such definitions shew the latitude of usage which the word enjoys. Useful as this elasticity may be in the literary world, it is fatal to psychology that aims at biological treatment of its material. This kind of "consciousness" would cover almost any kind of mental reaction whatever. The earthworm, in making a discriminative response, perceives (and so does the spinal cord) and could, therefore, be granted consciousness. At the other extreme, "totality of a person's thought and feelings" is just about equivalent to "personality".

Without spending any time in an aprioristic defence of my position, I will simply give the sense in which I intend to use the term, an endeavour in which I hope to be consistently successful. Consciousness will be the capacity of the subject to be aware of his thoughts as thoughts; the conscious person will be one who is not merely engaged in a mental reaction but is aware of that reaction as of something taking place within himself. In other words, it is something the existence of which the behaviourists either deny, or the utility of which as a concept they deny. Conscious mental processes will be such as are actively introspected or are dependent for their nature on that kind of examination (e.g. unconscious judgments in a case of submerged, secondary personality).

This statement may serve well enough as a delimitation of a certain field of mental phenomena; but that is merely negative. On its positive side it rests on the subject's testimony as to the inner events which he chronicles. He may be lying, he may be deluded, he may, as some behaviourists would say, be merely reciting a verbal formula that has been conditioned with some kinds of reflex behaviour. If introspection be our only source for scientific knowledge of consciousness, how are we going to deal with the problem as to whether animals have consciousness or not?

Or, in the field of psychopathology, how are we going to know whether a dissociated personality is conscious or not? Plainly we are badly in need of a description of the functions peculiar to consciousness apart from the data furnished by introspection.

I claim that I enjoy this peculiar endowment of consciousness and I believe this because I know that I "think". But how can I demonstrate that I have "thoughts"? The answer comes from everyday experience. We say that one person thinks about his work while another does it without thinking and we make this judgment confidently. The two types of behaviour must be different. The unthinking person responds either to an immediate stimulus or he responds to a definite remembered experience: in either case his behaviour is according to a set pattern. The thinking person, on the other hand, performs actions that are the response not to the environment alone, nor yet to discrete memories, but to some elaboration of the two that can have taken place only within himself. The thinking person can produce a truly novel bit of behaviour, adaptive to a new situation, while the unthinking subject does not. This formula is good enough for the layman, but "environmental situation" and "memory" are rather vague terms. It would be desirable to reduce this "thinking" to some simpler and more crucial data.

The simplest datum known to introspection is an image. If we can detect any reaction that could be determined only by some interaction of an image and consciousness, then we might derive therefrom an objective criterion of consciousness. If an image be merely a reproduction of a past stimulus, then it will operate as if it were a perception. That is, there will be a reaction, objectively seen, for which the image would be an appropriate response. If we are to stick to objective criteria, we should have no justification for saying that there was anything more than a repetition of the response; and, were it not for the subjective testimony of those who suffer from hallucinations, we might never suspect that there was any kind of a reproduction of the past stimulus. An anecdote related by William James[1] will illustrate this:

"I have observed a Scotch terrier, born on the floor of a stable in December, and transferred six weeks later to a carpeted house, make, when he was less than four months old, a very elaborate pretence of burying things, such as gloves etc., with which he had played till he

[1] *Principles of Psychology*, vol. II, p. 399.

was tired. He scratched the carpet with his forefeet, dropped the object from his mouth upon the spot, and then scratched all about it (with both fore- and hind-feet, if I remember rightly), and finally went away and let it lie."

There are, of course, two ways in which this behaviour can be interpreted. We might say with the behaviourists that it was a burying reaction conditioned with some visceral state that could be labelled as satiety; or we might ascribe subjective awareness to the dog. In the latter case we should have to call the reproduction of past experience an hallucination. The dog thought that he had a bone and that there was litter around him as in the stable. This example shews, I trust, that objectively an image does not function as a perception.

Now let us take another example. A few minutes ago I wanted to get the second volume of James's *Psychology*. I left my desk, walked to a certain book-case and glanced over the books on a certain shelf until my eye fell on the required object. What guided me to the correct spot? It was an image of the book in a particular part of a particular book-case. Had this image functioned as a perception, I should have never left my chair but reached up to grasp a purely imaginary book. Instead of that, the image excited a number of indirect responses, constituting a new pattern, that culminated in a perception identical in form with the image. Something told me that the image was an inner phenomenon and that to make it "real", to make it coincide with an external stimulus, I must get up and walk across the room. This something is consciousness.

It might be objected that here I am not really following the objective method because I have used introspective data. I would reply that an observer (unless he were a psychologist with a prejudice against images) could have deduced an image of the book from my behaviour. How else could the next example be accounted for? Koehler[1] reports that one of his apes, having

---

[1] *Mentality of Apes*, p. 136 seq. For data as to the behaviour of anthropoid apes I am going to quote Koehler exclusively. I do this not because I agree with his theoretic conclusions (which I consider as extreme in their way as are those of the behaviourists in the opposed direction) but because the internal evidence is convincing (to me) as to the unprejudiced control of his experiments, and because his observations are of just those mental capacities in which we are now interested. Furthermore, the reader will not have far to seek, if he wishes to read the full description of the experiments which I quote—an excursion he may find most entertaining.

learned to fit two tubes together to make a long stick, with which he might drag fruit within his reach, and being provided with a tube and a bit of narrow board, chewed at the end of the latter until he got it narrow enough to be inserted tightly into the tube. What could have guided such behaviour except an image *and* consciousness as I have defined them? The observation is the more noteworthy because this type of solution was rare in the problems which Koehler set his apes. In other words, the ordinary behaviouristic explanation of their exploits will hold for most of the data recorded. Occasionally, as in this incident, one seems to be forced to assume the existence of a reproduction of past experience that is discriminated from a perception and used as a goal *towards* which reactions tend rather than *to* which response is made directly.

With such examples in mind, we are in a position to frame an objective definition of consciousness. It is a capacity to discriminate between stimuli arising in the present environment and stimuli occurring as reproductions or elaborations of past experience. The discrimination is evidenced by the reproduced experience being utilized as a goal and not as a stimulus for an immediate and direct response thereto.

It should be noted that this definition does not imply that consciousness is a fixed and immutable faculty or function, that, having once appeared, remains unaltered during the further evolution of the species. It is, rather, a kind of function that marks a stage in evolution, one that can go on to higher and higher development with elaboration to include self-consciousness, utilization of abstract thinking, and so on. Like intelligence itself, it is something that has a gradual growth. This may not be the layman's, the metaphysician's, nor the ordinary psychologist's notion; and it is hoped that the reader may realize that I am using "consciousness" to cover a type of mental process to which he may have been giving some other terms or term.

CHAPTER VI

THE EVOLUTION OF INTELLIGENCE

WHEN an image is used as a goal rather than as an immediate stimulus, it may be said that *planning* takes place. In this we are bound to assume some kind of a prevision of an end and we are forced to this assumption by the demonstration of two phenomena: an immediate reaction to the "end" is inhibited and, at the same time, other reactions appear, which, in themselves, have nothing to do with the end reaction but are related to it only in so far as they may mediate the goal reaction. Evolution of intelligence is concerned with elaboration of preliminary reactions. The contrast between the pure stimulus-and-conditioned-response type of reaction and a somewhat more intelligent one may be brought out by two examples of behaviour of the same dog whose facility in forming conditioned responses I instanced in Chapter IV.

For the first eighteen months of his life he lived in the country during which period he saw a great deal of a chauffeur to whom he became greatly attached. Then he was moved to the city. The following performance was enacted innumerable times. He would see a car drawn up to the kerb with a chauffeur seated at the wheel. At once he would jump up to the front seat and sniff at the chauffeur, and then "register disappointment" as the cinema jargon puts it. To me, who knew his reactions well, this was the purest type of conditioned response. His capacity for visual perception was high, for he could recognize me at nearly one hundred yards' distance. But this stimulus liberated only one type of reaction, namely a dash in the direction of the person seen. The next element in the chain of behaviour was smelling; if it revealed an appropriate odour, then demonstrations of affections took place. (His dependence on smell for the exhibition of affection was shewn in another incident. I once came to his kennel accompanied by a much smaller man, a stranger to the dog, to whom I had loaned a fur coat of mine with which the dog was familiar.

For fully a minute he lavished his attentions on this total stranger, disregarding my voice and appearance, until he came near enough to me to get a really good smell. Thereafter he was indifferent to the stranger.)

Over against this futile type of routine response we may consider an incident shewing a higher degree of adaptability. When he was only three months old, I took him for a walk across some fields. At one point we came to a woven-wire fence; over this I climbed and then walked to a point some twenty-five feet from the path where a slight depression in the ground left a small space below the lowest strand of wire. I lifted up the wire and called to the puppy to crawl through, which he did. Two months later we covered this same ground for a second time. I climbed over as before and then waited to see what he would do. He made a brief and half-hearted attempt to get under at the point where I had crossed and then went directly to the depression twenty-five feet away. Here he made no attempt to crawl under but looked up at me and whined.

Our next problem is to reconstruct the probable stages in the evolution of intelligence between the initial stimulus and response level, where modes of reaction are rigidly fixed, and the level of specialized ability we call planning. Specifically, we seek to discover the steps taken in substituting indirect reactions for immediate responses and the increasing guidance of these by the desired end. These indirect reactions I shall call subsidiary ones, using this definition: A subsidiary reaction is one which is utilized as a step towards satisfaction of an appetite, although providing no satisfaction *per se*.

The first stage is the conditioning of a special series of subsidiary reactions to form a pattern adaptive to a new and specialized situation. Let us suppose that an animal wishes to get at some food—or other objective—but is impeded by an obstacle. Different species will behave in quite different ways. More stupid ones will try indefinitely to reach the objective directly. Others will soon cease the effort and indulge in more or less random movements in relation to the obstacle. If one of these succeeds, it will be attempted in a shorter time on a second trial and will eventually be integrated with the goal reaction and the specialized pattern will thus be formed. This type of solution is pure conditioning and its success rests (apart from innate facility for conditioning) on three possible factors, accident, training and the prior possession of the subsidiary reactions necessary for the composition of the new pattern. This last is the only one needing comment.

Koehler[1] reports that when hens are placed in a cul-de-sac closed by a grating through which they see food, they try in vain to get at it directly and when unsuccessful rush about in zig-zags. If in their wanderings they get to the end of the wall around which they ought to go, they make the detour. A dog, on the other hand, will make the detour almost at once. From this contrast it ought not to be deduced that dogs are necessarily more intelligent than hens; they probably are, but proof should rest on the solution of a large variety of problems that demand the exercise of differing types of responses. Dogs are hunters and, therefore, must be capable of approaching their quarry circuitously. The normal method of getting food in the hen is to wander about picking as it goes. Blocked in the effort to reach its objective directly, each species adopts an innate reaction that *might* solve the problem. The dog has a suitable response for this emergency ready formed; the hen has one that will succeed only by accident.

Another example from Koehler (p. 32) will illustrate this kind of solution in detail. Chimpanzees do not have to learn to use sticks as extensions of their arms; what has to be acquired is the application of this capacity to specific situations.

"Nueva was tested three days after her arrival....She had not yet made the acquaintance of the other animals but remained isolated in her cage. A little stick is introduced into her cage; she scrapes the ground with it, pushes the banana skins together into a heap, and then carelessly drops the stick at a distance of about three-quarters of a metre from the bars. Ten minutes later, fruit is placed outside the cage beyond her reach. She grasps at it, vainly of course, and then begins the characteristic complaint of the chimpanzee: she thrusts both lips—especially the lower—forward, for a couple of inches, gazes imploringly at the observer, utters whimpering sounds, and finally flings herself on to the ground on her back—a gesture most eloquent of despair, which may be observed on other occasions as well. Thus, between lamentations and entreaties, some time passes, until—about seven minutes after the food has been exhibited to her—she suddenly casts a look at the stick, ceases her moaning, seizes the stick, stretches it out of the cage, and succeeds, though somewhat clumsily, in drawing the bananas within arm's length. Moreover, Nueva at once put the

[1] *Loc. cit.* pp. 14, 15.

end of her stick behind and beyond the objective, holding it in this test, as in later experiments, in her left hand by preference. The test is repeated after an hour's interval; on this second occasion, the animal has recourse to the stick much sooner, and uses it with much more skill; and on the third repetition, the stick is used immediately, as on all subsequent occasions. Nueva's skill in using it was fully developed after very few repetitions."

In Koehler's fascinating study of apes marked discrepancies (from a human standpoint) appear between the advances made in different types of solution of the problems he set them. When a gymnastic exploit was possible their achievements surpassed the imagination of the experimenter. With "tools" held in the hand, their progress was considerable. On the other hand, their capacity to build was definitely limited. They could learn to climb on a box to reach an objective and even put one box on top of another in order to increase the height of the platform. But, in performing the latter feat, they were—humanly speaking—surprisingly stupid. No amount of trial and error seemed to teach them that it was difficult to balance a large box on a small one, or that a box would not stand on one corner. The property of bulk, or height, in an object seems to be the only one (if it is to be used in climbing) for which the chimpanzee has innate responses. Hence his "stupidity" in solving this kind of problem.

The prior existence of an innate response which might solve a problem may be invoked to explain episodic exhibitions of intelligence in animals who ordinarily exhibit no evidence of true images or of consciousness. Dogs, for instance, may occasionally perform feats that are most naturally explained by a human being with his introspective bias as true planning. If accomplished by a child, such an action is probably best explained as the result of conscious thinking, because man does use images and their utilization is at first episodic. But one should hesitate to account for an unusually intelligent act in a dog on any basis but that of his demonstrable capacities, until it is proved that these could not be adapted to accomplish the observed behaviour. If we bear in mind that a dog, when in an *impasse*, may reactivate an old reaction as a mere matter of trial and error procedure, we can explain some of its intellectual prodigies as lucky shots. If the same dog produced a variety of such solutions and did so consistently, the resuscitation of old reactions in trial and error would fail as an explanation.[1] Darwin[2] quotes two examples of "reasoning" that may be explained in the former manner:

"Mr Colquhoun winged two wild-ducks, which fell on the further side of a stream; his retriever tried to bring them over both at once, but could not succeed; she then, though never before known to ruffle a feather, deliberately killed one, brought over the other, and returned for the dead bird. Col. Hutchinson relates that two partridges were shot at once, one being killed and the other wounded; the latter ran away, and was caught by the retriever, who on her return came across the dead bird; 'she stopped, evidently greatly puzzled, and after one or two trials, finding she could not take it up without permitting the escape of the winged bird, she considered a moment, then deliberately murdered it by giving it a severe crunch, and afterwards brought away both together. This was the only known instance of her ever having wilfully injured any game'."

That both these incidents record intelligence must be granted. But that they necessarily exemplify reasoning is another matter. If frustration is going to cause the resurrection of an old reaction tendency, is there any more fundamental impulse in a dog than to kill its prey? The comment of a sportsman on these anecdotes is apropos. He told me that, if they had been his dogs, he would have beaten them, because there was such a danger of killing becoming a habit. The more intelligent behaviour in the second case would have been for the retriever to have carried the living bird in and then returned for the second, dead one. This might be an example of true planning and the possibility of its occurring in the first case is not to be dogmatically denied. The return of a hunting animal to its dead quarry is, however, an almost universal habit.

Apart from solutions like the above, which may be lucky accidents, the impression of intelligence, which animals at this stage of mental evolution certainly give, is due to facility in conditioning. Just before his retriever anecdotes, Darwin retails the following examples of this capacity:

"Rengger, a most careful observer, states that when he first gave eggs to his monkeys in Paraguay, they smashed them, and thus lost

---

[1] This might justify the exclusion by the behaviourists of "anecdotal" evidence. On the other hand, it must be remembered that some phenomena are, of their very nature, episodic. Should astronomers refuse to consider observations made on comets because these observations are not to be repeated at will? If we grant an evolution of intelligence, it is to be expected that its more specialized forms will appear, among intermediate species, episodically, just as a child, for instance, may furnish an example of true voluntary recall to-day and not repeat the feat for weeks.

[2] *The Descent of Man*, part 1, chap. 3.

much of their contents; afterwards they gently hit one end against some hard body, and picked off the bits of shell with their fingers. After cutting themselves only *once* with any sharp tool, they would not touch it again, or would handle it with the greatest caution. Lumps of sugar were often given them wrapped up in paper; and Rengger sometimes put a live wasp in the paper, so that in hastily unfolding it they got stung; after this had *once* happened, they always first held the packet to their ears to detect any movement within."

The intelligent solution of the fence problem by my puppy, as related above, is probably to be interpreted as an example of rapid conditioning and not of unequivocal planning. Prejudiced by pride of ownership, I regarded this feat for a long time as one ascribable only to true planning. But prolonged observation of him failing to reveal instances of unquestionable use of images, I am forced on the principle of parsimony to consider that he succeeded merely by using an old conditioned reaction. (His facility in this was extraordinary and led to his gaining a wide reputation for marvellous intelligence.) The crux of the matter is his whining and looking up at me. Was he asking for a consciously remembered assistance? Unfortunately this too is a habit reaction with most dogs who "appeal" to their master in any dilemma. Hunter, for instance, noted this occurring constantly with his dogs in the course of his "delayed reaction" experiments. Only the dogs did it; but in them the turning to the experimenter for clues seemed to militate against speedy learning of the required associations. In this case the experimenter never had assisted the dogs with the problem at hand, so the looking to him for a cue was a blind, "instinctive" action. But, considering the specialized adaptations of the dog to human society, it is easy to see how this kind of reaction is frequently successful—and, as often, flatteringly misinterpreted.

This, then, constitutes the first stage in the evolution of intelligence. The animal, when at a loss, produces old reactions more or less at random; one of these, if successful, is rapidly conditioned. A new pattern is thus formed and the animal is prepared to meet another similar situation more adaptively than he could before. This is preponderantly the type of intelligence in dogs, although I would not claim that they never achieve anything higher than this. How successful its development may be is evidenced by the utility of dogs to man. (Their mutual devotion is another story.)

The next stage in the evolution of intelligence is the *utilization of substitutes*. We have seen that the goal of development is the utilization of reactions that are chosen because they will lead to the realization of an imaged end. In the stage we have just considered, chance seems to be the dominant factor in determining the choice of the subsidiary reactions. The phase I am now going to describe seems to represent an intermediate level. When the objective is seen to be unattainable by direct attack, a programme of activity is inaugurated, that has been successful in the past, although the means for carrying out the programme are not obviously present. At the lower stage, the stimulus for the subsidiary reaction comes from the environment—an ape seizes a stick that is at hand and with it reaches out for some desired fruit. At the higher stage, the stimulus for the subsidiary reaction comes solely from the objective—the ape goes to look for a stick which is completely out of sight. At the intermediary level, the "stick reaction" is invoked, but some substitute is utilized that is at hand and which is used as if it were a stick. A banal example is the use by a bird in building its nest of some unfamiliar material when the customary material is lacking.

Koehler reports that his apes used in lieu of a stick stones, straws, old shoes, rags and so on. When the use of boxes, tables or ladders had been learned, "...stones, iron grills from the windows of cages, tins, blocks of wood, coils of wire, all these were indiscriminately collected and employed as ladders or footstools—objects which in the practice of chimpanzees are quite interchangeable". There are two conditions under which this procedure may result in a superior adaptation. The substituted object may serve the purpose of the reaction better than did that with which the activity was originally conditioned; or, occasionally, the object seized may elicit a reaction more appropriate to its nature. In either of these cases, new patterns are formed for the attainment of the desired end. The following quotation from Koehler[1] will illustrate the principles involved in the utilization of substitutes:

" ...after she had played with it a good deal, Nueva, for the following test, was deprived of her stick. When the objective was put down outside the cage, she at once tried to pull it towards her with rags lying in her cage, with straws, and finally with her tin drinking bowl which

[1] *Loc. cit.* p. 34.

stood in front of the bars, or to beat it towards her—using the rags—
and sometimes successfully.

"On the day after Tschego's first test, two sticks lay inside the cage,
about one and a half metres from the bars. When Tschego was let
into her cage, she at first stretched her arm out through the grating
towards the fruit; then, as the youngsters approached the coveted prize,
Tschego caught up some lengths of straw, and angled fruitlessly with
them. After a considerable time, as the young apes approached dangerously near the objective, Tschego had recourse to the sticks, and succeeded in securing it with one of them.

"In the next test, which took place several hours later on the same
day, the sticks were removed to a greater distance from the bars (and,
therefore, from the objective beyond them) and placed against the
opposite wall of the cage, four metres from the grating. They were not
used. After useless efforts to reach the bananas with her arm, Tschego
jumped up, went quickly into her sleeping-den, which opens into her
cage, and returned at once with her blanket. She pushed the blanket
between the bars, flapped at the fruit with it, and thus beat them towards
her. When one of the bananas rolled on to the tip of the blanket, her
procedure was instantly altered, and the blanket with the banana was
drawn very gently towards the bars. But the blanket is, at best, a
troublesome implement; the next banana could not be caught like the
first. Tschego looked blank, glanced towards the sticks, but showed not
the least interest in them. Another stick was now thrust through the
bars, diagonally opposite to the objective; Tschego took, and used, it
at once."

The modification of method occasioned by the nature of the
implement used is too obvious to deserve comment. Some interesting questions arise, however, from the apparent inconsist-
encies in the reported behaviour. If Tschego was clever enough
to "think" of her blanket, when it was not there, why was she so
stupid as not to use the sticks that were there? The answer is that
her getting the blanket was probably a random reaction. One
gathers that Koehler's apes used their blankets in a most indiscriminate way whenever they wanted any movable object. It is
important to note that a reaction conditioned originally with a
stick is transferred to a blanket, so that it becomes a "blanket"
reaction; the transition is so effective that sticks become inconspicuous! A stupider animal would look at nothing but sticks,
and would always perceive them, but he would not have the
versatility of potential intelligence.

These examples shew a strong tendency for the emphasis in
the subsidiary reactions to be shifted away from the environmental objects as stimuli and on to the general programme of

action. The question thus arises: What is the element in the environmental object which does serve as a stimulus? This is a problem that cannot be dealt with adequately until we have studied perception and meaning, but it must receive some attention at this point. At first "stick" is probably just an extension of the arm; i.e. it is something which can be grasped, and which provides sensory experience from its distant extremity, partly through touch but mainly through muscle, tendon and joint sense. All that is perceived is a solid, movable object; visual properties such as length and thinness seem to play a minor rôle, judging from the indiscriminateness of Koehler's apes. When the reaction of reaching out for something beyond the grasp is activated, the threshold is lowered for anything that can be grasped and manipulated. If the object now be used as if it had properties such as length and stiffness, which it does not possess, something occurs which is analogous to illusion in the human subject. When hallucination occurs, the stimulus arises wholly within the subject but is given external reference; in an illusion, one of a complex aggregation of properties is presented by an environmental object, while the others are internally elaborated and then projected on to the external object. We may say that the ape acts as if it had an illusion of a stick, when it really only holds a stone in its hand. In this "illusion" stage we see the beginning of what can be identified—objectively—as an image. When an animal responds to a stimulus that is externally non-existent, we say that an image —or image function—is present but is functioning as an immediate rather than as a goal stimulus, i.e. as an hallucination. When the essential nature of a reaction is determined by an internally elaborated something, (i.e. in the case of an illusion), this something is approximating the detached image function. By 'detached image function' I mean one that is operating as the stimulus to a new pattern and not one absorbed into a series of responses that make up an integrated pattern. The appearance of the illusion therefore represents an evolutionary advance, even though its exhibition may be non-adaptive, that is to say, of the pathological order. When a reaction is activated but needs an external stimulus to cause its complete overt expression, we speak of a liminal image of the external object lowering the threshold for the stimulus. When the reaction takes place without the presence of the external stimulus, an image function therefore is in operation. In the illusion phenomenon there is a mixture of these two imaginal processes.

The sequence of events in this case can probably be best outlined in terms of a specific example. An ape sees fruit that trial shews him to be beyond his grasp. Partially conditioned with this situation is the behaviour of reaching out for it with some implement. (Were the conditioning complete, an image function of the implement would appear that would either act as an hallucination or serve as a goal stimulus in the procurement of a real stick.) If, now, some object be at hand that can be picked up, the "stick" pattern, containing a liminal image of prehension, lowers the threshold for observing the object and it is picked up. This action then arouses the reaching-out-with-a-stick pattern to complete overt activity. The ape behaves as if it had a real stick in its hand. In other words, there are in operation image functions of such properties of a stick as the object does not possess. If the object be a stone, for example, there will be image functions of length, calibre, stiffness and so on.

It is in the substitution of image functions for the missing properties that the illusory, and non-adaptive, type of reaction consists. On the other hand, it is potentially an intelligent procedure, for if the image functions go on to the image stage and serve as goal stimuli, true planning may be achieved. This was accomplished by a number of Koehler's apes. Some of them made obvious attempts to manufacture missing properties as in doubling a handful of straws to give stiffness, or in stripping leaves from a branch to make it look like a stick. The manner in which most of the apes dealt with only one property at a time (such as stiffening the straw but shortening the bundle) shews what a gap there is between anthropoid and human intelligence. It is no feat for us to deal with all the properties of a stick—length, rigidity, calibre, weight, colour and texture—and to unify these into a unitary percept with such completeness that we are aware of any individual property only if it be absent or exaggerated. The ape has this capacity potentially in that he can produce image functions of one or more of them, but when these appear prematurely, before consciousness is there to deal with them, the illusion type of behaviour is exhibited.

Although it may be that adequate demonstration of the ape's capacity to react to properties appears only when these properties are obviously manufactured, yet the potential capacity is present earlier than this. If, placed in the predicament we have been considering, the ape is offered a choice of a number of objects that he can pick up, he will take a real stick, or the nearest approach thereto that his immediate environment offers. This justifies the view that the properties are represented already as liminal images. The origin of these is not far to seek. When the ape uses a stick, its properties determine integrated elements in the total "stick" reaction. Its calibre and texture will affect the way it is held; its weight and length the muscular effort used in wielding it; its length the coordination between eye and hand. Each one of these reactions involves the reception of tactile, proprioceptive or visual stimuli, or of combinations of these. When these specific reactions are excited in the absence of the stick, the sensory stimuli are reproduced as liminal images or as image functions, which are in turn representations of the "properties" of the stick.

If this term be taken to imply a reaction on the part of the ape to abstract qualities, it will be most misleading. Koehler offers very little evidence of the ape appreciating true abstractions. "Property" is simply a convenient shorthand label for a perceptual element that may produce a specificity in response. I may speak of the solidity of the table, for instance, when all that is in my mind is a feeling of incompressibility if I put my hand on it. Were I called upon to define solidity, I should, of course, introduce other experiences as well, all of them being generalized in terms of this property. The ape's recognition of a property is probably of this simple order. His "length" is not an extension in one dimensional space, but a feeling, vague and inaccurate very often, of "from here to there", as mediated by visual or proprioceptive stimuli. When he puts out his hand to grasp a banana, the extent of the movement is determined by the distance of it from his body. If distance determines his choice of, or search for, an implement to reach it, then "distance" is operating as a liminal image, or image. This is all I mean by "properties", but it should be pointed out that there is a further justification for the use of the term in the suspicion that analysis of *qualities* in the most advanced human sense is, perhaps, having its rudimentary beginning with the utilization of substitutes. If a certain pre-formed reaction pattern can only be expressed in the use of an object having some given property, then trial and error with substitutes will tend to isolate that property as a perceptual or imaginal stimulus.

It might be objected that there can be no such thing as a liminal image for a quality because threshold refers to quantity not to quality. If this objection were sustained, it would limit psychology to simple physiological experiments. A prime characteristic of mental reactions is the response to qualitative difference. The point at which a quality can be discerned constitutes its threshold, and it is impossible to express this in purely quantitative terms. Liminal images, therefore, represent the operation of past experience in facilitating responses to stimuli having less quantitative-qualitative value than those stimuli with which the reactions were first conditioned.

The impetus for utilization of substitutes comes from appetite, that is an activization of patterns fundamental for the survival of the individual or species, the organization of which we shall be examining in the next chapter. The dynamics of this type of behaviour come, then, from an appetite, but there is always an environmental stimulus which acts as a final objective. If the latter be materially absent but the same kind of conduct is observed, we speak of it as *Play*. Common to the behaviour I have called utilization of substitutes and to play is the application of reactions to inappropriate, or inadequate, objects, the treatment of them as if they were something else. The biological purpose of these exercises seems to be the practising of the reactions in question, for they seem, in each species or variety, to represent appetites, interests or adaptations fundamental for the type of animal. Dogs, for instance, play at fighting, hunting, killing small animals, and at coitus. The terrier tribe will add to this digging—in quite inappropriate places. The play of apes is vastly more extensive, while in man its range is almost limitless.

In higher animals, such as apes, the utility of play may not end with mere practise of useful reactions. An object manipulated in play may engender reaction patterns appropriate to its specific nature and these may later be utilized to solve real problems. In man, of course, it is impossible to say where play leaves off and research begins. A good example of the evolution of useful patterns in the course of play is seen in the history of the "jumping-stick" as related by Koehler.[1]

[1] *Loc. cit.* pp. 71, 72.

"Jumping with the aid of a pole or stick was invented by Sultan, and first imitated, probably, by Rana. The animals place a stick, a long pole, or a board upright or at a slight angle on the ground, clamber up it as quickly as possible with feet and hands, and then either fall with it in some direction, or swing themselves off from it at the very instant that it falls. Sometimes they spring to earth again, at other times on to a grating, beams, the branches of a tree, etc., often to a very considerable height. [Use of the pole as if it were a tree.] And at first it is certainly not circumstances that 'forced the leap upon them'. They could have 'got there' much more easily by walking or climbing. Also the landing-stages they selected seemed to offer no special attractions, so that when we take into account the constant repetition of this performance, we can only conclude that it is done out of the wish to *jump and leap per se*, just as children walk on stilts 'for fun'.

"But soon this form of play developed into the regular use of a tool. Sultan made the attempt to reach the objective (in the course of an experiment) in vain, as it was hung too high for him. He leaped straight into the air from the ground several times, and in vain; then he seized a pole that lay in his vicinity, lifted it as though to knock the prize down, and then desisting, pressed one end of the pole into the ground beneath the objective, and repeated the 'climbing jump', as above described, several times in succession. His movements had a certain playful and sketchy character, as though to say: 'It won't be any use!' and it was not. On the next occasion he was more resolute and more fortunate; he approached a solid piece of plank, so heavy that he could only just cope with it, placed it in position and started climbing and jumping off. Three observers who were present maintained that he could not possibly reach the objective in this manner, and on three occasions the treacherous plank fell over before he could swing himself away, but on the fourth trial he succeeded and tore down the fruit."

It is, perhaps, in the playful utilization of substitutes that we can discern the germ of what is to become *imagination* in the human being. We detect this not merely in the fact that the goal stimulus is not actually present. The unreal nature of the objective permeates the whole train of actions; they are not performed with the completeness seen in subsidiary reactions that tend towards material achievement. Puppies scuffle with one another; they do not bite deep, the dog worrying a rag does not try to eat it; the football player—if he "plays the game"—does not wilfully injure his opponent.

When imaginations are carried over into real life they may be either futile, silly, insane, or they may provide useful new solutions for previously insoluble problems. Discovery and resourcefulness begin with the utilization of substitutes as the achievements of

Koehler's apes with the jumping-stick shew. (Inventiveness belongs rather to the next stage.) The "insanity" of using substitutes without the procedure being controlled by images and consciousness was exhibited many times in the same animals. For instance, Koehler describes[1] how Rana, who could never learn to use a stick properly as an extension of her arm, would not try to knock down fruit with sticks suitable for such a method of getting it, but would try endlessly to use them as jumping-sticks, even when they were so short that she had to bend over to get her hands on the top of them. The folly lies in reaction being made to isolated properties.

The next stage in the development of intelligence is the *Combining Tendency*. So far we have noted only two ways in which previously separate patterns are integrated together. In one, the stimuli for the patterns have occurred consecutively in the environment a sufficient number of times for conditioning to take place. In the other, a substitute has been utilized whose nature has modified the subsidiary pattern concerned therewith: the total pattern has thus become modified and is, in effect, a new combination. In both these types, the bringing together of the unit patterns is dependent on environmental influence. Correlated with this is the rôle of the image functions, which have served solely to unite patterns already integrated together (except when their operation has been maladaptive). We now come to the consideration of combinations that are effected *via* images and in independence of specific environmental influence.

Let us suppose that some objective, such as food, has been successfully approached in the past by two well-integrated chains of reactions. In each case the last action in the series has been the same, *viz.* the actual seizing of the food. A new situation arises in which either reaction alone is inadequate, so that the animal is placed in the predicament which tends to bring out its latent capacities. So long as the food itself acts as a stimulus, it can only activate one reaction series. But, if the seizing of the food be imaged, and this image (or image function) serve as the goal stimulus, then both chains may be evoked together, i.e. they may be combined. So long as no consciousness is operating to control the combination, the order may be $a \to b$, $b \to a$, or they may be

[1] *Loc. cit.* p. 129.

carried out together as *ab*. Trial and error will decide which one of the three is most suitable. As a matter of fact, true planning is usually present if the intelligence of the animal be high enough to admit of the combining tendency. Accident may, however, be the deciding factor as the following examples from Koehler[1] shew. In these tests the chimpanzee had, in order to get a stick with which to reach for some fruit, to move a box to a point from which by standing on the box he could reach the stick. The apes were accustomed, of course, to reaching for food with a stick, and to moving and climbing on boxes—but the latter reactions were conditioned only with the last acts of food-getting. One of the chimpanzees, Koko, started repeatedly with the box, as if to bring it near the stick, but each time had to pass by the fruit, which then distracted his attention. He once used the box as a stick and succeeded; another time he put the box as near to the fruit as possible and then climbed on it. Eventually, he solved the problem correctly and, having done so, repeated the performance without trouble—the proper combination was integrated. (The attraction of the ultimate goal causing a break-down of an apparently planned action is analogous to the substitution in human beings of automatic for intelligent behaviour in an emotional crisis.) The next example shews a regression from the combination method to the utilization of substitutes (twice over), a probably accidental solution of a difficulty and, finally, achievement by the original, and correct, method:

" . . .the box is filled with stones. Sultan looks around for a moment, notices the stick on the roof, gazes at it concentratedly, goes to the box, and pulls it with all his strength towards the stick. As he can barely move it from the spot, he bends down and takes out one stone, which he carries under the stick; he places the block upright against the wall, but after one look up, he does not climb it after all.... Thereupon he at once drags the same stone to the bars opposite the end objective, and tries to push it between them; obviously the stone is to be used as a substitute for the stick. But, although otherwise practicable in shape and length, it will not go through the bars. The rest is clear and simple: Sultan again turns towards the box, takes another stone out, with difficulty pulls the box (still weighed down with two blocks) under the stick, stands it upright (whereupon the last stones accidentally fall out), takes the stick down, comes to the bars with it, and immediately reaches the objective."

---

[1] *Loc. cit.* chap. VI.

The combining tendency seems to be a specialization of the higher animals. It is rarely, if ever, observed in such animals as dogs, but permeates the play of children. Since a moment's reflection will bring many nursery instances of it to the reader's mind, human examples may be omitted. Its occurrence among chimpanzees is, however, worthy of citation.[1]

"Nueva was especially ingenious. Having once discovered that it was possible to dip water out of the butt with her little drinking cup, she incessantly dipped and filled the cup and then poured back the water into the butt. She hardly drank it at all, but even the drops that ran down the cup were of interest to her, and she loved to dip her hand into the water and watch the rain of drops fall from it. She also used her bread—for which she did not care very much—in this water game; she dipped and soaked it and then sucked the water from it; dipped and soaked again, and so forth. [This is, perhaps, mainly the utilization of substitutes, but not the following where no accident can have brought the elements together.] She was also an indefatigable 'collector'. She scraped together stones, pieces of wire and wood, rags and banana skins, into heaps on the ground, into her nest, or into a tin bowl, and seemed to derive the greatest satisfaction from the procedure. None of the other animals had so developed a taste for collecting and putting objects together. Three days after her arrival in Teneriffe, she split a wooden plank with her teeth and drove a wire into the gap; on the following day she was busy with a woollen rag which she tied to a stick; she was not content with simply wrapping it around the stick, but actually achieved a sort of knot, by looping one end of the rag through the portion wound round the stick and pulling it taut. However humble this effort may seem to the general public, it has an amazingly *constructive* character for anyone who knows the tearing, smashing, and demolishing tendencies of the species. Other apes than Nueva also liked to poke about with straws (or sticks) in holes and crevices, but I never observed any of them 'weaving' and carefully plaiting straws through the wire interstices as she did. She had a special fancy for knots; for instance, she thrust a strip of banana leaf through a wire mesh, laboriously drew the end back through another mesh, tied the two ends together, and continued in the same way, either by slipping one end of the leaf through the knot, or tying the ends again. I often thought that she was about to begin a deliberate, though rudimentary, constructive effort, a form of manual craftsmanship, but she never could be induced to continue these efforts on any plan, however easy. When I prepared for her a wooden frame with a few loosely inserted strips of leaf, she turned aside and devoted herself to her own knots; the slightest pressure towards anything stable and 'productive' extinguished her joy and interest at once, and she let the frame fall in sullen displeasure."

[1] Koehler, *loc. cit.* pp. 323, 324.

This paragraph describes two correlated features of the mental life of chimpanzees that are of prime importance for our present scheme. (Nueva was, of course, an unusually intelligent animal, but her achievements differed more in degree than in kind from those of her fellows.) Not only is the capacity exhibited of uniting modes of behaviour, which have not been conditioned together by environmental accident, and therefore establishing new relationships between objects, but this combining tendency seems to be followed as an end in itself. To the outsider, it appears as if a new and specific "instinct", or rather appetite, had been developed —a driving force similar to, although not so powerful as, hunger, self-preservation, or sex. The status of play in the hierarchy of instinctive processes is a matter to which attention will have to be given later on; but it must be pointed out now that the pursuit of combination as an end in itself must have profound influence on further intellectual development. We have here the germ of "intellectual pleasure" that is so important for human culture. Nueva was inventing, for the sake of inventing, and we know that in great human inventors the lust for new combinations often takes on a truly compulsive character.

Another type of combination remains to be discussed. Koehler reports a number of instances where a correct reaction for the solution of a problem was adopted, but where the means at hand were insufficient. In this emergency the chimpanzees sometimes attempted to make good the deficiency through duplication—a sort of vague reaction to the property of quantity and, we might therefore say, a beginning of arithmetic. The duplication may take the form of addition of another tool (chosen indiscriminately), or there may be an inappropriate combination of right tools, or an ineffective combination of right tools. As we saw with the utilization of substitutes, the tendency is to react to one property at a time and not to synthesize various properties—a method demanding conscious manipulation of images. Here the reaction is the property "inadequacy", and the response to this is just "duplication". As a result of trial, error and accident, correct solutions may, however, be achieved, and thus a new tool manufactured. Then manufacturing becomes a new subsidiary reaction. The story of this achievement is truly exciting, but would take too much space to quote in full. Some of the data should, however, be mentioned.[1]

[1] Koehler, *loc. cit.* chap. IV.

Chica, when she found that her stick was not long enough to reach the objective, repeatedly took a still shorter second stick and held the two end to end in her hand. Having thus made a stick that was optically longer, she went on fishing for her fruit with the new stick in spite of the foolishness (from a human standpoint) of her effort. Similarly Rana, wanting to reach some fruit with a jumping-stick, would put two little sticks end to end, covering the join with one hand. She then actually tried to climb up this optically longer rod. Sultan was set the task of reaching food placed outside the bars of his cage and beyond the reach of any single stick. His sticks were hollow bamboo rods of varying calibres, so that it was possible for them to be jointed together like a fishing rod. The steps he took in finally achieving a jointed stick that would work are extremely instructive.

First he tried to use one stick and then the other. This failing, he dragged a box up to the bars, but then pushed it away again without using it. He next pushed out one of the sticks on the ground in the direction of the fruit, and then propelled it further with a second stick. With some patience and dexterity, he managed thus to touch the coveted object, and this seemed to give a temporary satisfaction. After a while this achievement palled, and he left off his experiments without the end-to-end position of the two sticks having, apparently, suggested the insertion of one into the other. He seemed at this point to abandon all thought of getting the fruit, but a short time thereafter began to play idly with the two sticks. In the course of the play, the two sticks happening to come into line, he shoved one into the other and started off for the objective with his new, elongated stick. When, the joint being loose, one stick dropped out of the other, he kept replacing it, until he managed to rake in the fruit. "The proceeding seems to please him immensely; he is very lively, pulls all the fruit, one after the other, towards the railings, without taking time to eat it, and when I disconnect the double-stick he puts it together at once, and draws any distant objects whatever to the bars." The next day he pushed one stick with the other towards the food for a few seconds only, then adopting the jointed stick technique with facility. Two weeks later he managed, after some trial and error, to make a triple-jointed rod. Two months later he achieved a triumph of tool-making, for he chewed down the end of a board until it was small enough to be inserted into the end of a bit of bamboo rod.

Before leaving the discussion of the combining tendency two possible implications of it for human psychology should be mentioned. It is possible that what some psychologists and sociologists have called the "constructive instinct" in man is simply the combining tendency given human expression. The other has to do with a process fundamental in psycho-analytic theory. The combination principle makes possible the integration of patterns previously quite distinct. Different patterns may thus co-operate towards a common end. This—or so I have argued[1]—is the fundamental principle in sublimation.

The last stage in the development of intelligence is true *Planning*. I call it the last because I believe that the type of mental process involved in the simplest example of planning is the principle operating in the highest achievements of the human intellect. Whether or not the method should have the same label when its material is abstract thought is a question of taste, or of expedience, which need not concern us now.

In true planning the choice of means, and of the subsidiary reactions belonging thereto, is not arrived at by actual experiment; the experiment is carried out in imagination, so far as that is possible, and the means thus chosen are then applied in actuality. By imagination I mean the treatment of images by consciousness as images. The possible means to the desired end, the attendant subsidiary reactions, are represented as images to a functioning consciousness: the principles of random choice, utilization of substitutes and combination present various solutions to consciousness in imaginal form; the effects of the imagined behaviour are also produced as images and these are compared with the situation as actually perceived. If judgment declares that a certain imagined course of action can be executed successfully, then—and only then—do the images become stimuli for overt behaviour. In other words, trial and error is carried out in imagination. It is to be well noted that the function of consciousness, according to this scheme, is critical rather than creative. The creative elements come from utilization of substitutes and the combining tendency, both of which functions seem to have incorporated with them some kind of an instinctive or appetitive urge. This view is in harmony with the introspective testimony of

[1] *Problems in Dynamic Psychology*, p. 357; *Psychology of Emotion*, p. 187.

creative thinkers who claim that their ideas "come to them"; they are not elaborated directly by voluntary, conscious effort.

A simple example may clarify the principle involved in planning. I come to a woven-wire fence and want to get across it. Automatically variant solutions come to mind: I might jump over it; but it looks beyond my agility. I might climb over; but I see barbed wire on the top which might tear my clothes, moreover the horizontal wires look as if they would sag and furnish a hazardous foothold. I might crawl through, so I look for a gap but none of the meshes are large enough. I might crawl under, and look for some depression in the ground, but none deep enough is discovered. I decide to vault over and this I do after first having picked out the solidest-looking post on which to place my hands. Had I the mind of a rat or a dog, the likelihood is that I should have made all these trials in actuality and probably sustained bodily injuries, not to mention the damage to my clothes. Being human, I have merely moved my eyes and carried out all the trial and error in imagination, a process lasting only a few seconds, involving no risk, and saving much energy.

Now this account is made up from memories of many such experiences and so may be taken, I presume, to be accurate so far as it goes. If so, the absence of still further modes of dealing with the situation are interesting in that they throw light on the probable origin of the imagined solutions. I did not think of moving any object near the fence which might serve as a platform from which to jump. This is because the situation I visualize is an empty field; if, however, I were faced with this problem and there were a box lying near, I should certainly think of using it. One stimulus for the imaged solution is, therefore, the environmental presence of an implement that might be used. The sight of the top, meshes, and bottom of the fence probably play some rôle in summoning the images of climbing over and of crawling through or under. If I now begin to cudgel my brains to think of other possible solutions, I imagine the use of wire-cutters and pole-vaulting. But these are arm-chair fabrications. In a real situation, it is extremely unlikely that they would ever come to mind; in fact, I am aware that I imagine rather another person than myself surmounting the obstacle in either of these ways. This is because they are not habitual methods for me. To a soldier on the Western Front, or to a pole-vaulter, they might be natural fancies. The conclusion is that imagined solutions are those already conditioned with similar problems or arise as responses to environmental stimuli. In either case their appearance is automatic. Granted a sufficiently critical consciousness, the degree of intelligence exhibited in any bit of planning will rest on the wealth of potential reactions already present and on the capacity of the subject to inhibit actual trial and error procedure. Associated with the latter is the capacity to maintain attention on the problem until a sufficient number of images of possible actions to include an expedient one has arisen. It is thus that the "will" to solve a problem becomes an important factor.

The necessity for the prior existence of a subsidiary pattern that might solve the problem is a condition that cannot be too strongly emphasized. The reports that Koehler gives of the various achievements of his chimpanzees shew a striking irregularity—that is from a human standpoint. When success depended on agility and fine muscular co-ordination, they might reach a goal by a route which human judgment would eliminate as impracticable. In using sticks, etc., they shewed not only manual skill but true imagination and resource. On the other hand, their capacity in utilizing solid objects on which to climb, including the piling of boxes on top of each other, was limited. As Koehler says, their use of statics was physiological rather than psychological; that is, they could balance themselves but not external objects. A human being would judge that, once an ape had learned to move a box in order to climb up on it, he would have no difficulty in moving it if it happened to be in his road; yet the reverse seems to be true. The same animals, that had become accustomed to collecting boxes to stand on, failed for a long time to reach objectives when all that was necessary was to shove the box aside. It seems as if the box could be perceived as "movable footstool", but not simply as "movable". The bear—a much stupider animal—would probably knock the box out of the road without hesitation, because moving large objects is a routine reaction with him (lifting logs to look for grubs).

Once the combining tendency is developed, another source of subsidiary reactions is opened up. I have mentioned that I can imagine someone else vaulting over a fence with a pole. If imitation can operate through images, the range of potential subsidiary reactions is greatly widened. This is a capacity that is probably unrepresented below the human level. Chimpanzees, for instance, can directly imitate each other, or they can—at times—image their own procedures; but Koehler presents little or no evidence to indicate an imitation *via* images. This origin for subsidiary reactions introduces a social factor in intellectual advance. If the method of getting round a difficulty arrived at by one man can be applied to another difficulty by a second man, the advance of culture becomes cumulative. This principle accounts for the extraordinary acceleration in the advance of technical science which has characterized the last century. An example in point is the recent improvement in the phonograph. "Broadcasting" produced a technique for the production of sound through variations in an electric current. This knowledge was taken over by the phonograph manufacturers and translated into mechanical terms with astounding results.

There remains to be discussed the rôle that consciousness plays in planning. We human beings, who are so familiar with images as introspective data, may be apt to take consciousness for granted and fail to realize how maladaptive images would be if they were not under some kind of critical control. Our recognition of images as images is so constant and our foresight of the ends of imagined behaviour so facile, that we are likely to be unaware how close in mechanism is the solution of a problem by planning and the reaction to hallucinations. Yet, when consciousness is weakened (as in a variety of diseased conditions), the combining tendency leads at once to delirium and, in animals with rudimentary consciousness, images turn into hallucinations except under favourable circumstances. Koehler devised one test that could only be solved (in the first instance) by unequivocal planning and, although a number of his chimpanzees were able to solve it, their mistakes were all traceable to this tendency.[1]

The front of a cage was closed with bars through which the animal could see fruit lying on the floor beyond its reach. At the back a board was removed at a greater distance from the ground than the length of the ape's arm. Behind the cage was a stick tied so that it could only be used from behind. In order to get the fruit, it was necessary for it to be poked towards the front of the cage and then for the animal to run around and pull it out by hand. This meant that in addition to combining several subsidiary

[1] *Loc. cit.* pp. 263 seq.

reactions together in a novel order, an image of action from the front had to determine the direction of moving the fruit. If this image acted as an hallucination, it would simply result in futile efforts to grasp the fruit prematurely; consciousness had, therefore, to hold this image as an image, that is, as a goal towards which subsidiary reactions tended, and not allow it to function as an immediate stimulus. All the chimpanzees tended, no matter how well they began, to regress to a pulling rather than a pushing movement with the stick. That is, they tended to move the fruit at a direction of 0° rather than at 180°. The effects of distraction of consciousness on this part of the procedure are beautifully shewn in the following quotation:

"...in the next experiment, *from the very beginning, the direction towards the bars is clearly taken.* There is no doubt that this is the beginning of the solution. But now occurs one of the strangest performances that I have ever noticed in these animals. During the board experiment Chica had already frequently turned off from the right track (180°) and, for moments, reverted to the primitive direction (0°). While working now perfectly correctly and clearly towards the bars opposite, she is startled by a noise from the street, looks for an instant towards the scene of the disturbance, and then continues her activity, *but now pulling at* 0°; this time the change is *not* corrected. Chica continues pulling until the objective is brought close up to her under the wall with the gap; and *at this moment, like someone who has nothing more to do than to reap the fruits of his efforts, she runs round the cage to the bars*; nobody could look more nonplussed than Chica, when she peered into the cage and saw the objective as far as it could be from the bars."

The peculiar function of consciousness is well illustrated in this example—where it failed. For planning to be successful, it is not merely necessary that the goal should be imaged and a combination of subsidiary reactions oriented towards this end. The relation between the image and the subsidiary reactions must be maintained and *this relation exists only in consciousness*. So, when consciousness lapses, a combined reaction may go on, but a well-integrated, habitual, subsidiary pattern takes the place of a novel one. The goal image is still there, but, having lost its orienting function, it becomes a mere hallucination—as poor Chica discovered to her dismay!

We see thus that intelligence, of a human order, demands the presence and co-operation of three factors: first, the necessary unit reaction patterns must be in existence; secondly, it must be possible to combine pre-existing patterns *via* common images; thirdly, a stable consciousness must be present, which can correlate a goal image with the combined subsidiary reactions oriented to that end. Clinical observation would indicate that the feebleminded are much like chimpanzees in their mental endowment. The first qualification is not lacking; but the second is limited and the third episodic and flickering.

These defects are brought out in a test for feeblemindedness that I have found useful in preliminary examination. It is the more instructive in that I have found even advanced dements to pass it with ease. The material used is an ordinary watch with hour, minute and second hands and a stop-watch with a centrally mounted second hand. Nowadays, everyone is familiar with timepieces, so the subject matter of the tests contains no element of disconcerting novelty. It is found that the really low grade cases can only read the superposition of hour and minute hands as "dinner-time", and the vertical 180° position as "supper-time". Most of them can tell the time at five-minute intervals, but that is the limit of set reactions even among quite high grade cases. After that point, telling the time becomes a matter of reasoning. Suppose the hands are set at 18 minutes to 3. The patient calls it "a quarter to three". When urged to give the exact minute, the chances are even whether he will say "twelve minutes to three" or "eighteen minutes to three". He can add and subtract such small numbers with facility, he knows the principle of radial movement and he knows "to" and "after". Moreover, he can, under pressure, combine them, but consciousness is not developed up to the point of choosing one combination rather than another. To the question, How far does the minute hand travel when the hour hand moves three little spaces? he may give a series of pure and ridiculous guesses. This is a matter not settled by observation and memory, for he has never watched a clock long enough to see the event take place. He has to image the two movements and correlate them. The correlation comes from conscious critique, and here he fails. A comparison is next attempted between the ordinary and the stop-watch. He is asked to say what sort of time the big hand on the stop-watch tells. His answer is prompt and invariable: it is a minute hand. Even when he is asked to pick out the hand on the ordinary watch that travels at the same speed as the second hand of the stop-watch, he makes the same error; he compares the latter to the minute hand. There are three properties of a watch hand by which it is identified, its position on the dial, its size and its speed of rotation. To an intelligent man, the last is the all important one, for with him telling the time involves the formation of a new pattern by combination of the data derived from the absolute positions of the hands and corre-lated by a conscious use of the knowledge of relative movement. The feeble-minded subject acts according to the behaviourists' rules. He has a set of "times" corresponding to a series of absolute positions of the hands. These are determined only by the size and location of the hands. He is not totally without the knowledge of radial movement, but this property sets up no reaction which he can correlate with those stimulated by the other properties of the hands. For him, therefore, the generalization "time" does not exist, for he knows only a limited series of "times". It has often been said that the essential defect of the feeble-minded lies in their incapacity to deal with abstractions. This analysis arrives at the same conclusion but reduces the defect to terms of simpler mental processes.

To anyone familiar with the feeble-minded, the reading of Koehler's book brings up a clinical parallel with almost every page.[1] The chimpanzee is so proficient in the reactions he has learnt—even quite complicated ones—he is so like the well-trained but stupid workman who performs his routine task with admirable accuracy but who fails so strikingly when the situation demands some change of method involving imagination. In fact, the whole argument of this chapter could have been written around data gathered in the observation of human defectives, just as well as on the basis of Koehler's inimitable study of chimpanzees. The one real advantage of the latter material is that it is, biologically, normal, and hence not open to the criticisms so facilely directed against pathological evidence. That such criticisms are based on ignorant prejudice is, from the standpoint of expedience, irrelevant.

This chapter may well be brought to a close with a brief dis-cussion of an example of "planning" drawn from the life of Pasteur.

[1] For a discussion of this subject and extensive references to the literature, see Lindemann, Erich: "Untersuchungen über primitive Intelligenzleistungen hochgradig Schwachsinniger und ihr Verhältnis zu den Leistungen von Anthropoiden", *Zeitschr. f. d. ges. Neur. u. Psych.* Bd. 104, S. 529.

It is suitable for analysis, because the problem and data are simple, while at the same time its results were momentous.[1]

In 1847, Pasteur turned his attention to a problem that had interested him for some years. It was that of the relationship of crystal structure to the polarization of light in solutions of the crystals. The data he had at hand were a general knowledge of crystal forms and two specific bits of information. John Herschel had shewn that solutions of asymmetric crystals rotated polarized light one way or the other so that a correlation was established between the right- or left-handedness in crystals and the right- or left-handedness of rotation of polarized light in their solutions. The other specific fact was that some crystals, apparently homogeneous, could be seen under the microscope to be a mixture of crystals with differing symmetries.

The problem arose from a note made by Mitscherlich and read by Pasteur three years before to the effect that the tartrate of sodium and ammonium, although identical with the paratartrate of sodium and ammonium in all other physical and chemical properties, differed from it in rotation of polarized light: the tartrate was dextrorotary while the paratartrate was neutral. Why these otherwise identical substances had differing effects on polarized light was the question that kept recurring to him. "I could not understand that two substances could be as much alike as Mitscherlich said without being identical."

Occupied with this query, Pasteur was looking at some tartrates under the microscope when he observed that they had tiny facets on the corners too small to be seen by the naked eye and so previously overlooked. At once he formulated an hypothesis by combining Herschel's discovery with his own observation. The tartrates might be really right- and left-handed, although the facets which shewed this were microscopic, while the paratartrates were perfectly symmetrical. So far, except for the recondite nature of the subject matter, this is no greater achievement than the combination for the first time by a chimpanzee of climbing on a box and reaching for some fruit with a stick. Consciousness had still to play its part and it was here that Pasteur's genius was demonstrated. This imaged solution had to be tested against actuality.

[1] The best account of this work which I have read is in *Pasteur and His Work*, by L. Descour, chap. II. My data are drawn from it, and from it I shall quote. If the reader be unfamiliar with the terms used, he can find them explained there.

"All of a sudden I was filled with emotion. The great surprise which Mitscherlich's note on the tartrates and paratartrates has occasioned me, had always remained. In spite of his very careful study, I said to myself, of these two compounds, Mitscherlich cannot have perceived that the tartrate is dyssymmetrical, as it should be; nor can he have seen that the paratartrate is not, which is equally probable. At once, with feverish activity, I prepared the double tartrate of sodium and ammonia, and the corresponding paratartrate, and set about comparing their crystal forms; with the preconceived idea which I had just formed, of dyssymmetry in the tartrate, and the absence of dyssymmetry in the paratartrate form. Thus, thought I, all will be explained; Mitscherlich's note no longer will be mysterious; dyssymmetry in the form of the tartrate will correspond to its optical dyssymmetry; the absence of dyssymmetry in the paratartrate will correspond to the absence of activity of this salt on polarized light, to its optical indifference. I discovered, in fact, that the tartrate of ammonia did bear facets betraying dyssymmetry; but when I came to the crystalline form of the paratartrates I had a momentary shock, for all these crystals bore dyssymmetrical facets."

Here was trial demonstrating error. At this point, an ordinary intelligence would have resigned the problem. Pasteur did not. The goal image of crystal difference, to which he tried to make reality (by his procedure) correspond, was not abandoned, but a new composite image was fabricated by utilizing the other bit of specific experience—that some crystals shew variation of symmetry under the microscope, proving the substance to be really heterogeneous. This stimulated another series of reactions. He scrutinized the paratartrate crystals closely and saw that there was a mixture: some had right-handed facets and some left. Laboriously—although feverishly—he separated them, and then dissolved the separated masses. To his joy he found that one group rotated polarized light to the right and the other to the left. The paratartrate was optically neutral because it was a mixture of dextro- and laevo-rotary substances! It has been said that the modern science of physical chemistry descends from this experiment. Yet it differs from the planning of the chimpanzee only in that the method which the poor ape (and most men) follows half-heartedly and falteringly is, by a genius, pursued relentlessly and consistently.

The consistency, one might think, comes from the more or less mechanical and static functions of combination and conscious critique; but the relentless pursuit smacks of something emotional, dynamic. We have already had occasion to note that there may be a lust for utilization of substitutes or for combination pursued as ends in themselves: whether we call this play or not, it has to be admitted that some driving force is at work in the practising and perfecting of intellectual specializations. In the case of Pasteur, why did he not give up his problem when his first hypothesis fell to the ground? Why, indeed, did he ever have such an insatiable curiosity about the correlation of crystal structure and optical properties? This leads us over to our next problem, that of appetite and interest.

CHAPTER VII

APPETITE AND INTEREST

PATTERN reactions, as we have so far discussed them, have been essentially responses to environmental stimuli, although we have also considered the mode by which some of these stimuli may become represented internally. Instincts are patterned reactions of this order, and yet we know that, in frequent usage, instinct is held to be the directing agency in behaviour that is not initiated by any external stimulus. For instance, both layman and psychologist will say that a good deal of human behaviour is traceable to the sex instinct, although a very large part of this occurs in the complete absence of a member of the opposite sex. We see, then, that we use the term instinct to cover the seeking of a stimulus as well as the response to it. More critical psychologists make a discrimination between these two types, calling the former appetite rather than instinct.

How do we judge, objectively, that an appetite is in operation? We observe an animal apparently searching for something: if now we translate "searching" into terms of stimulus and response, we must say that the animal exhibits a low threshold for a certain group of environmental stimuli, and a heightened threshold for others. For instance, the hungry animal hunts, and we presume that he is hunting because we see him relatively indifferent to any stimulus except that of food. There is, then, a goal towards which a train of reactions is tending although this goal may not be objectively evident when the train is set in motion. The stimulus for this programme of behaviour may come from the actual presence of the goal (e.g. food), or it may originate in a visceral disturbance. It is in this latter case, where the programme is initiated by something within the organism, that we have a right to speak of appetite.

It is possible to account for the transference of the initiating stimulus from an external to an internal source on the assumption that the latter represents a conditioned response—the conditioning having taken place, of course, during the lifetime of the species rather than of the individual. Originally (but only in the lowest animals), we may assume that the only stimulus was actual food. When this was swallowed (or ingested), complicated visceral reactions took place; in time, these became integrated with the food-getting reactions. In animals that eat periodically, there are metabolic swings. That is, after eating and digesting food, there is a period during which fuel and tissue building substances are being stored up and, following this, as consumption goes on, there is a deficit of such substances in the general bodily economy. This deficit is present when the animal eats again, hence the re- actions of digestion may have been integrated with the katabolic ones. Since digestion has followed regularly on eating, and eating on food getting, the whole series may have been conditioned together. When the total chain is thoroughly integrated, any one of the elements may be represented by an image function. Cannon, for instance, has shewn that in hunger there are actual rhythmic movements in the stomach analogous to those that occur when food is present there. In other words, the hungry animal acts as if it had taken food into its stomach. The result of this complicated integration would be that katabolism would lead to digestive image functions and these, in turn, to a low threshold for external stimuli of food. We can see, then, how the integration of food- getting reactions with visceral disturbances, could produce just such a lowering of threshold for a goal stimulus as is seen when appetite regulates the behaviour of an animal.[1]

Although we may reconstruct the origin of appetite in this manner, there remains to be considered an analogous directing agency in human behaviour, in which neither the actual stimulus is present nor is it possible to demonstrate a visceral disturbance of sufficient intensity to account for the "drive" exhibited by the

---

[1] It might be objected that quite lowly organisms shew reactions to be fairly described as appetitive. We must bear in mind, however, that any such recon- struction as this is artificial. It is probably impossible to find any animal with any definitely organized serial behaviour that does not exhibit at least rudi- mentary appetite. In fact, if we look on an appetite as merely a chain of reactions that may begin with a visceral disturbance rather than with an environmental one, the very organization of an animal that gives it its specific existence as an organism would have something appetitive in it. In other words, pure stimulus and response is probably a hypothetical unit convenient for the physiologist, but never existing actually in an unmodified form.

The biological implications inherent in the claim that conditioning can be affected through a series of generations is a matter to be discussed in Part II.

individual. For instance, it is a simple enough matter to say that
the love of a man for a given woman is at bottom sexual, but it
notoriously exists in the material absence of the woman herself—
it may persist even after her death—and this devotion may still
be strong after the sex glands have atrophied. Psychologically
the impulses remain, although physiologically their stimulus has
ceased to be. These peculiar appetites are to be properly labelled
interests.

If we grant the dependence of appetites on visceral disturbance,
we may derive interests from appetites by a somewhat similar
process of progressive conditioning, bearing in mind that in man
the presence of an active combining tendency makes possible
elaborations of patterns that would be impossible in lower organisms. When an appetite is in operation, there is a lowered
threshold for an environmental stimulus, that is to say, there is a
liminal image of the goal. If the integration of the chain of reactions
proceeds still further, the liminal image may become an actual
image or image function. We see this in various physiological
manifestations, as, for instance, salivation with hunger, prostatic
secretion, erection, etc., in libidinous excitement, or goose flesh in
fear. These manifestations do not quiet the original visceral
disturbance and there then results either a general restlessness, as
is common among the lower animals, or an imaginal activation of
more patterns—that is, the unsatisfied appetite inflates the combining tendency. Very often, of course, there is a combination of
these two phenomena. The second type is naturally a response
of more highly organized creatures but, if they be so organized,
it is just as inevitable an occurrence as the vague reaction of
restlessness.

This throws a little more light on the problem of *play*. Play
serves two purposes: it gives an outlet to weak excitations set up
by weak visceral disturbances, and it facilitates the integration of
new patterns, as we have seen in the last chapter. When the intensity of play reactions is increased by the augmentation of the
visceral disturbance, the restlessness phenomenon intervenes. Or,
if the environment offers the goal stimulus in actuality, there is an
expression of the patterns in their normal intensity: the play
becomes real.

Unsatisfied appetite leads, then, to an exercise of the combining
tendency to more and more patterns being activated imaginally

and integrated together. If this process goes on long enough, if a given appetite be often enough aroused and not satisfied, an ever-enlarging system of imaginal gratifications may be built up. The greater this elaboration the wider will be the range of stimuli and responses that are integrated in this secondary and purely imaginal system of patterns. This means that the environment is more and more likely to duplicate elements in the imaginal sequence. When this occurs, there is an opportunity for overt response to a real stimulus and the underlying appetite may thus gain some satisfaction. It is not direct, it is true, but if it occurs often enough it may succeed in quieting the original disturbance. In time, this superstructure of the appetite will become integrated with the secondary stimuli and so a relative independence of the visceral initiation may be thus achieved. This superstructure I have elsewhere[1] called "an instinct-motivation". If consciousness be directed to this constellation of imaginal patterns, *fantasy* is recognized.

A translation of the foregoing argument into terms of introspection may make it more understandable. If a man be stirred by some appetite and the means for its satisfaction be not at hand, he begins to imagine how his goal might be achieved; that is, there comes to his mind the various methods and their circumstances by which satisfaction has been gained in the past. The original process in these imaginations is planning. In the development we are now considering, the planning is not successful in attaining the final goal, but there is a realization of some reaction associated with the goal. For instance, a man desires possession of a woman, weaves fantasies about her which include such possession as is possible. This may be only the handling of some trinket of hers, but it gives a partial satisfaction. This may—under appropriate circumstances—become an end in itself, and is then known as fetishism:

> "Schaff mir ein Halstuch von ihrer Brust,
> Ein Strumpfband meiner Liebeslust!"

> "From her breast for me a kerchief fashion,
> A garter be my love and passion!"

If the sight of the fetish will now excite the total system, the stimulus has ceased to be visceral, and the complex has become an instinct motivation rather than an appetite.

---

[1] *Problems in Dynamic Psychology*, p. 260.

Such development is characteristic of man, but its beginnings may be seen lower in the evolutionary scale. I have already cited an example of this in Koehler's chimpanzee Sultan. When he succeeded in making his double jointed stick, he gathered in fruit—and inedible objects as well—apparently for the "fun" of mere gathering. In the ape, such an instinct motivation is larval, for the crude appetite breaks through, before any large elaboration of associated patterns is well integrated. This may be, in part, due to his rudimentary consciousness being unable to gain satisfaction from images, that is, such imagination as he can compass is used in planning, he gets no pleasure from fantasy as such.

The higher the organization of an animal, the more complicated do its instinct motivations and their combinations become. This has two effects: First, more potential experience is included in the images or image functions; and, therefore, the environment will offer more stimuli capable of activating the motivations. Second, the greater the complication of this system, the more impossible is it for any environment to duplicate all the images, that is to satisfy the motivations in actuality. There thus arise in a creature so highly organized as man, programmes of activity that are for ever progressive, and these are *interests*. The environmental stimulus may arouse and allow overt expression to a unit pattern in this large integration. But if this means the imaginal activation of the whole series, a disturbance of the appetitive order is created anew, and this leads to a further exercise of the combining tendency —or, to put it in introspective terms, to further fantasies of satisfaction.

The more highly organized is any creature, the larger will interests bulk in his life, and the more independent will they be of primitive patterns connected with visceral disturbances. This means that in creatures with a large combining tendency there will be a practically constant flux of imaginal pattern reactions, that will proceed so long as the central nervous system is physiologically active. This flux—usually quite unconscious—is the basis of the kind of "mind" which is studied introspectively.

It may be noted here, that this hypothetical reconstruction of interest is applicable to psychopathological, as well as to psychological, theory. It is seen that the essential conditions demanded for the development of interest are: (1) a stimulation of patterns of primitive biological importance; (2) a failure of the environment to provide opportunities for overt expression of these patterns; and (3) the existence of the combining tendency. This view rationalizes modern psychopathological theories, in the foreground of which stands psycho-analysis. According to Freud, the frustration of the sexual appetite leads to an unconscious elaboration of fancied satisfactions. During the war the same, or an analogous, mechanism was demonstrated in connection with fear. When that was aroused, fantasies of dangers and of escape from them were often so elaborated as to constitute the chief interest of the soldier, which led in time to his incapacity with a neurosis. The primal instinct most generally and consistently frustrated in civilian life is the sexual one, which justifies the stress that has been laid upon it; both theoretically and practically, however, all kinds of personal ambitions may suffer the same kind of blocking and secondary unconscious elaboration in fantastic satisfaction.

These considerations introduce a perplexity as to nomenclature. We can hardly speak of the danger reactions of anxiety states constituting "interest", for inherent in that term, as ordinarily used, is the notion of something consciously desired. Yet, from an objective standpoint, the exhibitions of unconscious pre-occupation with danger are like those of pleasurable ones. I will, therefore, use the term "pathological interest" to denote the unconscious processes that eventuate in symptoms, since their mechanism is identical with those culminating in the conscious programmes properly called "interests". In this way, the confusion may be avoided that has been engendered by the Freudian term "unconscious wish", which is so often an ambition abhorrent to consciousness.

It should further be noted that this account implies that interests are essentially irrational. As a matter of fact, it is the very failure of fantasy to correspond to environmental reality that makes the building of interests progressive. Of this Pasteur gave an excellent example. The genius formulates fantasies which refuse to fit in with the herd theories that are applicable only to a small range of facts. He, therefore, seeks other facts which may duplicate elements in his fantasy (discovery), and continually modifies his fantasies (hypotheses), adapting them to the wider range of facts.

In more highly organized beings, mental activity is probably always going on during waking life, and, perhaps, during much of sleep as well. This activity is a flux of images having three sources of initiation,—external stimuli, proprioceptive stimuli, and images of both of these, aroused by association, and proceeding in directions controlled by interests. In civilized man, the third type of stimulation is by far the most important. Over this vast chaos of potential thoughts and actions broods consciousness, continually selecting what shall emerge as introspectively known thought. The interactions of consciousness with this basic flux produce the various phenomena that have been artificially divided by psychologists into "faculties". These must now be examined briefly.

CHAPTER VIII

ATTENTION

THE behaviour of an organism relative to an object can, for purposes of analysis, be divided into three phases, of which at least the first two are always present. At the outset, there is an orientation to the stimulus which we call attention; then comes a generic response, appropriate to the nature of the object, which is called perception; finally, there may be a specific response peculiar to the setting of the object, either in the environment or in the past experience of the individual, this last constituting meaning.

The simplest of these three is *attention*. It is complicated for introspection by the recognition of at least two types, voluntary and involuntary. In the latter, attention is *drawn to* the object, while, in the former, it is *directed towards* it. With voluntary attention there is an awareness of conation, purpose, effort. It is, therefore, not simple: there is the relationship between subject and object, called attention, which follows a willing process that produces the relationship. This relationship is orientation towards the object preliminary to the specific reaction to it. The object may, of course, be something environmental, proprioceptive, or a thought.

This orientation may be observed in the experimental production of conditioned reflexes. Beritoff[1] conditioned various stimuli with a flexion reflex in the fore limb of a dog, in response to a painful stimulus of that limb. He found that the flexion of the limb has a conditioned response developed after two to six combinations. As a rule, associated conditioned reflexes of the head, in the form of an orientation reaction, were obtained before the conditioned reflex of the limb. In other words, before the response "It hurts", there is behaviour which betokens "Something is going to happen there", although there is nothing in the experiment to indicate

[1] "On the Fundamental Nervous Processes in the Cortex", *Brain*, vol. XLVII, p. 120.

true consciousness. The organism is merely thrown into an expectant attitude.

The non-voluntary type of attention may be divided into two sub-types, automatic and coerced. The former is an unwitting reaction to objects in the fringe of consciousness, while, in the latter, the object seems to compel the subject to a conscious recognition of its existence. We have, then, to deal with three types of orientation reactions, voluntary, automatic and coerced attention. Both the non-voluntary ones can be treated as threshold phenomena: that is, the threshold is lowered for the object, and raised for other objects. Since these are simpler phenomena than those involving volition, it would be better to consider them first. The fundamental problem is what determines the threshold.

We may take the case of *automatic attention* first. It might seem as though an environmental stimulus merely excited automatic and unwitting responses in an organism that was quite neutral to the stimulus prior to its appearance. For instance, if a man is walking down the street, he avoids other people *when* they appear. But it may be shewn that many patterns of orientation operate without active awareness in such a situation. This is evident from the fact that we can find our way to an habitual destination without any conscious effort or awareness that we are making any choice between the various sets of landmarks to which we must be responding selectively. Some orientation patterns are, therefore, active in every such instance. On the other hand, these orientation patterns may be definitely inhibited, as is seen in "absent-mindedness". If a man, walking along the street, concentrates his attention sufficiently on some train of thought, he will not only bump into other pedestrians but may actually lose his way. Another proof of the existence of these automatically operating orientation patterns is that different systems of orientation obtain with different modes of progression. The pedestrian, the cyclist and the motorist respond to different kinds of environmental stimuli. Similarly, we may have temporary development and disappearance of specific susceptibilities. During the war, when I was in uniform, I became instantly aware of the insignia worn by other men in uniform; now, if I note anything, it is simply that a given passer-by is in uniform, his rank has ceased to have any significance.

The determination of a response by a pattern subliminally activated may be demonstrated in the course of conditioned reflex experiments. Beritoff[1] working with the flexion reflex to a painful stimulus found that at first there were many accessory reactions, such as groaning, howling and writhing. These diminished in the course of the conditioning until there was no objective movement except that of the flexion of the limb stimulated; but he found that a repetition of weak electrical stimuli, not producing anything externally visible except a weak flexion, would so lower the threshold for these accessory reactions that the conditioned stimulus then applied would produce marked groaning, writhing and howling.

Some important facts in relation to attention appear in the phenomena of absent-mindedness, which, as we have just seen, is really a matter of inhibition. The success of many conjurors' tricks depends on a sedulously invoked inattention. A friend of mine has given me an excellent example of this. He watched a street performer throw a stick up into the air where it disappeared. Then he left the scene, but turned round again at a distance of about 100 feet. As there was an opening through the crowd, he could still see the conjuror apparently repeating the feat. This time, however, he saw the performer very clearly place the stick behind his back. At that distance, he was unable to hear what the conjuror said, or perhaps to follow with his eyes the slight movements which served to distract the attention of those close at hand from the real manipulations with the stick. The acme of "absent-mindedness" is reached in the somnambulic stage of hypnosis, where the subject responds to—and is apparently aware of—only such stimuli as he is ordered to attend to by the hypnotist, with the result that he is apparently insensitive even to deep pinpricks. There is seemingly, in the activation of patterns, a high selectivity which is artificially controlled. But the matter does not rest there, for, parallelling the exclusion of intercurrent stimuli, there may be an incredible lowering of threshold for suggested responses. For instance, a subject may respond to the sound of a pin dropped on the floor in the next room when the doors are closed. This shews that there is a reciprocal relationship between the thresholds for the selected and the excluded patterns. That is, inhibition of the irrelevant is correlated with facilitation of the relevant. This inhibition is not necessarily conspicuous in normal life, although inevitably to be deduced from the phenomena of

[1] *Loc. cit. Brain*, vol. XLVII, no. 3, p. 372.

attention; but, when it amounts to the total anaesthesia of the somnambulist, it cannot be overlooked.

We can, therefore, say that in automatic attention there is an activation of patterns so habitual as to perform their function at the fringes of consciousness, and so adequate in their operation as not to need the kind of modification which is accomplished by full consciousness. The development of automatic from voluntary attention is in evidence whenever a game is being learned. For instance, a good tennis or lawn tennis player moves to the correct position for receiving the ball before his opponent even strikes it. At the beginning, he has to learn painfully that a given posture of his opponent means that the ball will be directed in a given direction. Later on, he gets to respond to this posture without any conscious awareness of what he is doing.

Coerced Attention. Here the stimulus breaks in on and interrupts current behaviour or thoughts. Naturally, any very powerful stimulus, such as a flashlight or an explosion, will activate some pattern totally irrelevant to the programme of behaviour that has been in progress. This is too obviously a matter of threshold to deserve any discussion whatever. Under this heading, however, we must consider both the normal phenomenon of distractability, in which an apparently inadequate stimulus breaks in on a train of thought or behaviour, and the abnormal phenomenon of compulsive thinking. In the latter, the patient is plagued by the eruption into consciousness of totally irrelevant and often quite painful thoughts. The genesis of these has been studied in different schools of psychopathology and the same conclusion reached as to their origin. It has been found that these troublesome thoughts are only parts of "complexes". The complexes are prepotent unconscious patterns the activity of which may be demonstrated by hypnotic technique. Repression prevents the appearance in consciousness of the whole complex, but is not strong enough to prevent some portion, or representation of it, from coming into awareness. In a certain way, therefore, the activation of these unconscious patterns is like that of the automatically operating orientation patterns we have just been discussing. In both cases, some pre-existent stimulus has set going a system of patterns (such as the reaching of a given objective) that determine reactions without the intermediation of consciousness. In the pathological case, however, no exercise of will can ever bring the complexes as such into consciousness, whereas the orientation patterns in normal life may come into full awareness if there be the slightest desire to inspect them. Unconscious mental processes that are active but cannot be brought into consciousness have been termed co-conscious by Morton Prince. The psychopathological example shews, then, that compulsive thoughts do not come from nowhere, are not accidental, but are exhibitions of pre-activated patterns.

Distractability seems to be due to two factors, chance and a waning of conation. The second is certainly a factor and will be considered partially under voluntary attention, and more fully much later on when we have occasion to study fatigue.[1] If we were without leads from psychiatric observation and without technique developed in psychopathological work, we should probably have to rest content with the statement that chance may determine distractability. In various psychoses, however, particularly mania, patients are constantly commenting on things in the environment which are apparently trivial. We have already seen in studying free associations that these comments are not accidental but are determined by an underlying trend, that is to say, by an active series of patterns important in the unconscious mental life of the patient. Similarly psycho-analytic investigation of the same phenomenon in normal people may shew precisely the same determination.[2] We may conclude, therefore, that in coerced attention the reaction to apparently trivial stimuli is due to the activation of patterns of which the subject is not aware. These principles are nicely shewn in one of Koehler's experiments:[3]

"Chica did not come to this solution though the stick was hung in position in her presence (April 23rd) and also touched and moved in order to attract her notice. (May 2nd): The stick was again fastened to the roof while Chica looked on. She took no notice of it, but tried to reach the fruit with a flaccid plant-stalk, and then to tear a plank loose from the lid of the box; finally she tried to reach the fruit with a straw. Then she appeared to lose interest and began to play with her companion Tercera; the stick seemed no longer to exist for her. Suddenly some one in the distance called loudly; Chica started and looked round, and, in so doing, caught sight of the stick. Without any hesitation, she went towards it, leapt straight upwards twice, and unfortunately for the purposes of investigation, succeeded in reaching it, as a slight rise in the ground assisted her efforts."

[1] In a subsequent book.
[2] See *Psychology of Emotion*, pp. 241–2.
[3] *Loc. cit.* p. 184.

In this observation we see four stages in the development of attention: (1) no attention is paid to the stick whatever; (2) "stick patterns" are activated by using straws; (3) totally different behaviour is instituted; (4) attention is distracted from the latter by the sight of the stick. If we were to put this sequence in terms of human psychology, we should say that unconscious stick patterns had been activated to the point of becoming co-conscious, and that these had then finally determined attention to the stick.

Voluntary Attention. The naïve view is that voluntary attention is an active process in which conscious volition determines the extent of what is perceived. A little reflection, however, will shew that this can hardly be true, because everyday experience teaches us that the type of life of any given subject will determine very largely the range of what he sees or hears. For instance, a North American Indian, while walking through the forest, will see the tracks of animals that are invisible to a European and still inconspicuous to the latter when they are pointed out to him. We are also most of us familiar with the necessity of having a front seat in the theatre when a foreign language is spoken; we may be able to follow the play but only when the sound stimuli are more intense than those we need for an understanding of our own language. Susceptibility for certain perceptions may also be acquired through training; for instance, a European after sufficient study may be able to detect the "tones" in Chinese which no amount of voluntary effort could lead him to discriminate before this study. Similarly, a painter trained in anatomy will see the elevations and depressions on the skin of his subject caused by underlying muscles, whereas the anatomically innocent painter cannot observe them. These data would indicate that the rôle of volition is merely to activate one pattern, or a group of cognate patterns, and that it is the latter which then determine the threshold for that which is perceived. This principle is experimentally demonstrated in the "Aufgabe" experiments, where conscious prevision not only facilitates a given performance but makes others more difficult.

According to this view, then, volition cannot affect the threshold directly but determines attention merely by the activation of patterns, which in turn operate as in coerced attention. I have demonstrated this in a number of subjects with a very simple experiment. As all stamp collectors know, there are very faint

marks on some stamps which are called plate numbers. I shewed
such stamps to a number of people, telling them what they
ought to see. Some—both collectors and non-collectors—who
had extremely good vision were able to detect the numbers with
the naked eye. But most of them could not see the numbers
unless they had first observed them through a hand lens. Once
this had been done, however, the perception could be repeated
with unaided vision. This was true even of one subject who was
a collector and thoroughly familiar with plate numbers. The
orientation in this case probably consisted in getting the numbers
into the centre of the visual field.

Consciousness, it appears, operates only in voluntary attention
and then its operation is to regulate the choice of patterns, as a
rule, rather than to control the pattern directly. The question as
to how consciousness performs this feat is not one that can be
discussed at this point, since it involves more factors than we have
already in hand. We may mention, however, that the selection of
reaction patterns is a function of personality; in fact personality
is demonstrated in this choice. From this it follows that voluntary
attention will increase with the development of personality, and
that where personality reactions are weak, attention will be more
of the coerced type. This latter is apparently true of children. So
long as their personalities are undeveloped, without the establishment of dominating interests to cause a selection of patterns, the
environment will impress itself on the child with greater evenness,
and hence there will be response to a larger number of details.
This is shewn in *eidetic imagery*.[1]

This is a peculiar phenomenon which has recently been observed in
many pre-adolescent children. The subject is handed a picture, for
instance, and told to scrutinise it for a short time. The picture is then
removed, and he is instructed to look at a neutral background and
visualise the picture that he has seen. When true eidetic imagery is
present, the child seems able to construct an incredibly detailed reproduction; for instance, he may be able to count the pickets in a fence or
discover in the image other data that would be impossible for an adult
to recollect. There is no evidence adduced to shew that any great complexity of detail may be reproduced a long time after the real object is
seen, provided no immediate reproduction has been demanded. It is,
therefore, probable that we are dealing here with a simple memory of
the immediate past, at this age not yet transformed into ideas and word

[1] Probably the best account in English of this subject is to be found in a
paper by G. W. Allport in the *Brit. Jour. Psychol.* vol. xv, no. 2.

memories. From an individual standpoint this is probably as useful—so far as concrete experiences go—as are verbal and ideational memories; but, being relatively incommunicable, eidetic imagery can have little value in social adaptation. In an artist, however, communicability being possible through the pencil or brush, eidetic imagery might remain a socially adaptive capacity. With the establishment of dominating interests, only patterns consonant with these interests are easily activated, hence there develops a greater selectivity of details attended to *pari passu* with the specialisation of interests in the developing personality. This means that the adult will have a lower threshold than the child for certain stimuli but that with this there will be an active inhibition for the irrelevant environmental data to which the child responds with facility. Whether the child or man is the better "observer" depends entirely on what one considers good observation to be. Under certain circumstances, naturally, the maintenance of eidetic imagery in adult life may be of real advantage as the following quotations from Taine[1] will shew.

"An American friend of mine, who has this faculty, describes it to me in these words: 'When I am in my corner, facing the wall, I see simultaneously the chess-board and all the pieces, as they were in reality after the last move. And as each piece is moved, I see the whole chess-board with the new change effected. If I am in doubt in my mind as to the exact position of a piece, I play over, mentally, the whole game from the beginning, attending carefully to the successive movements of that piece. It is far easier to deceive me when I watch the board than otherwise; in fact, when I am in my corner, I defy any one to mislead me as to the position of a piece without my afterwards detecting it....I see the piece, the square, and the colour, exactly as the workman made them—that is, I see the chess board standing before my adversary, or at all events, I have an exact representation of it, and not that of another chess board. So far is this the case that, before retiring to the corner, I begin by carefully looking at the chess board and men as they stand, and to this first impression I mentally attend and revert'. Usually, he does not see the table cloth nor the shadows of the pieces, nor the minute peculiarities of their make, but can recall them if he wishes."

"An English painter, whose rapidity of execution was marvellous, explained his mode of work in this way: 'When a sitter came, I looked at him attentively for half an hour, sketching from time to time on the canvas. I wanted no more—I put away my canvas, and took another sitter. When I wished to resume my first portrait, I took the man and sat him in the chair, where I saw him as distinctly as if he had been before me in his own proper person—I may almost say more vividly. I looked from time to time at the imaginary figure, then worked with my pencil, then referred to the countenance, and so on, just as I should have done, had the sitter been there—when I looked at the chair I saw the man'."

[1] *On Intelligence*, pp. 38, 45.

The discussion of attention may be thus concluded: Attention is a state of preparedness to perceive. This preparedness consists in the activity of one pattern and a reciprocal inhibition of others. But, so long as the process does not go beyond the point of mere attention, the patterns are not fully activated; were they so, overt behaviour or subjective perception would take place. We must, therefore, conclude that the flux of image functions, constituting the patterns in question, are not in full play, but that they have been aroused only as liminal images. Our formula would therefore be: *Attention is the activation as liminal images of certain patterns, which thus produce a selective orientation towards certain stimuli.*

CHAPTER IX

PERCEPTION

AFTER attention orients a creature towards any environmental object, a sensory phenomenon known as *perception* takes place. This is true whether the perception be a subjective cognitive experience, or be deduced from the observed behaviour of the creature. The second condition being simpler will be considered first.

We say that a cat perceives a saucer of milk because its behaviour is appropriate to milk; it does not indulge in indiscriminate muscular contractions, such as might ensue from a sudden strong olfactory, visual, or tactile stimulus. We, therefore, conclude that something in "milk" has elicited a certain set of patterns. We know of no cognitive process in the cat and, indeed, if there were such, it could not correspond accurately with the environment, for the cat's conduct is instinctive, that is to say it follows set patterns. The occasion for the reaction is something set up in the cat by the visual stimuli proceeding from the saucer and milk. It involves images as we have seen, or at least, image functions, that is, past experience operating somehow in the present. So far as we can tell, the cat perceives nothing for which it has not already some potential specific response. If we were not introspective, we should think only of reactions and probably never speak of perception at all. Objectively, then, perception is a name for the process in the cat which activates a certain reaction pattern when a given stimulus is applied.

But the case is not quite so simple as this. Were it so, the cat would begin to make drinking movements without first approaching the milk; moreover, it approaches it accurately. This means that more than milk is seen and responded to. There are proprioceptive stimuli from the eye muscles and there are attendant image functions aroused by sight of the floor on which the saucer rests, and so on. In other words, the perception involves not merely an activation of generic reaction patterns but also of orientation patterns, whose image functions give a *penumbra* to the central image. Thus, a correct direction for the response is secured or, to put it in sensory terms, the perception is properly localized. The existence of a penumbra differentiates a perception from an image objectively.

When perception occurs there is, subjectively, an awareness of the process which is projected on to the stimulus. One might think that there was a direct mental representation of the stimulus, were it not notorious that experience really determines what is perceived. Roughly, we see or hear only what we have seen or heard before. Of course, we may perceive new combinations of known elements, but we only perceive details in a complex that we can identify. Subjectively, the past experience recurs in image form. A stimulus activates certain patterns: if these result immediately in overt conduct, there may be no subjective perception (automatic behaviour), but, when consciousness is directed towards the process, there is an awareness of the images belonging to the patterns. But if this were all there would be no external reference and little correspondence between the object and the perception.

Both of these arise from what I would call *background* phenomena. Let us consider the visual case. The object perceived is not the only thing that sets up images; innumerable other visual stimuli enter at the same time and each of these activates its own image or images. When an image in the focus of awareness is attended by a penumbra of other images with which it stands in a certain relation, it is given external reference and called a perception. This relationship is a peculiar one: in the first place, attention is focussed more on the central image; and, in the second, the central image blocks out a bit of what would otherwise be a continuous background. For instance, a book which I perceive rather than merely imagine excites my attention more than does the table on which it rests, while at the same time the table is incomplete. The images composing my subjective appreciation of it have a gap where the book lies.

These conditions are fulfilled with dreams and hallucinations. The things seen have background on which they are superposed and part of which they exclude. The external reference which a true hallucination enjoys is due to the fact that it is apparently related to the environment as is a true perception. Hysterics and other favourable subjects, in whom hallucinations can be produced artificially, all declare that the imaginary object comes in between their eyes and the furniture of the room. For instance, one hysterical patient of mine was frequently accompanied by a sabre-toothed tiger. This animal would come in the door and lie down on the carpet, part of the carpet then becoming invisible to the patient. If I walked across the room, she would have to check herself to keep from calling out a warning to me lest I should trip over the beast. An image, however, has none of this background: if I see a book not on a table, shelf, floor, nor held in someone's hand—in other words, not causing a gap in my visual field—I call it an image. This is a judgment, a function of consciousness, and I suspect that the faintness of the visual experience of an image, which so many psychologists have attempted to allege as discriminating it from a true perception, is really a product of this conscious judgment. The vividness of eidetic imagery in children may very well be due simply to the relative weakness of their partially developed consciousness.

Assisting in the formation of the background of perceptions there are naturally images of other senses. For instance, one may touch the object seen, there are proprioceptive stimuli from the eye muscles, and so on. The rôle of these accessory images is too obvious to demand more than this mere mention of them.

With true perception the process is, therefore, not simple. The stimulus arouses an image, or group of images, specific for the object, and there is then a reference back to the object and its background, the final perception resulting from the correlation of the original image and the penumbra images. This process probably accounts for certain phenomena observed in conditioned reflex experiments.[1] When first formed, a conditioned reflex is "generalized", that is, any stimulus analogous to the conditioning one will produce the conditioned response. (For example, if touching one point of the skin is the stimulus, a later stimulation of distant parts of the skin will elicit the same reflex; or, if a musical note be the conditioning stimulus, a wide range of notes will be also effective in producing the response.) The conditioned reflex may, however, be differentiated. In this process, widely differing stimuli (e.g. high and low notes) are used, one being "reinforced" by following it with the appropriate stimulus for

---

[1] "The Irradiation of Conditioned Reflexes", G. V. Anrep, *Proc. Roy. Soc.* B, vol. XCIV, 1923, p. 407.

the inborn reflex, while the other is not so followed. The latter
will soon cease to elicit response. Then another pair closer together are similarly discriminated until, finally, only a very small
range of conditioned stimuli will be effective (to within half a
tone for musical sounds). This is like an "accurate" perception
—it is produced by a "reference back" that confirms the presence
of the inborn stimulus in one case and denies it in the other.
When there is no discrimination, the conditioned reflex is said to
be irradiated or generalized.

If reference back is impossible, differentiation of a conditioned
reflex cannot be secured. This state of affairs exists with the
"trace reflex", i.e. one produced by giving first the conditioned
stimulus and then, after a pause, the inborn one, so that there is
no overlapping of the two stimuli.

"These reflexes, even when finally established, remain fully irradiated, so that at any time a stimulation of any spot on the skin will
produce a salivary secretion identical with the secretion obtained by
stimulating the spot originally used for the formation of the reflex.
The reflex will be equal in force and will have the same latent period
whatever spot of the skin is stimulated. The irradiation of trace reflexes
with a long latent period (long pause between the two stimuli) is even
wider than this. They irradiate over the boundary of the tactile receptor
into the areas of other receptors. So that, although the initial trace
reflex was formed with a tactile stimulus, an application of heat or cold
to any spot on the skin will produce a similar reflex. Moreover, the
irradiation of these reflexes does not confine them to the skin only but
penetrates into the areas of the distance receptors—auditory, visual, etc.,
so that, if a dog has a firmly established tactile (or any other) trace
conditioned reflex with a long latent period, a stimulus applied to any
of the receptor organs will cause a secretion of saliva which will have
the same latent period as the original reflex, but will be somewhat
smaller in quantity."

Normally, this reference back is performed so quickly that there
is no awareness of it; it is really part of the continuous waking
orientation that was discussed in the last chapter as automatic
attention. But if the background be difficult to examine, or time
be too brief for adequate re-examination of the background, faulty
perception may result owing to the maintenance of the first and
central image to be excited. This was shewn very nicely in some
experiments by Bartlett.[1]

[1] "An Experimental Study of Some Problems of Perceiving and Imaging",
Brit. Jour. Psychol. vol. VIII, part 2, May 1916.

He exposed pictures of complicated scenes in a tachistoscope. The subjects with repeated exposures (up to fifty and more) stuck to their original, and often false, interpretation, and added more and more false details to substantiate the interpretation.

I once suffered from an interesting illusion to be somewhat similarly explained. I was sleeping in a room, that had a door at the end of the wall against which the head of the bed was placed, so that while lying on my side I could just see the door by raising my eyes. I woke one night and, on opening my eyes, saw what seemed to be a muffled light moving slowly from the door to the middle of the room. I interpreted this instantly as the passage of a burglar with a covered light and sat up in bed with the words "Who's there". But, before the words were well out of my mouth, I realized what I had been looking at. In a straight line from my head to the door, there was a clock with an illuminated dial resting on a bed table. The dull glow from this had provided a visual stimulus; but, in the absolute darkness of the rest of the room and in my position of muscular relaxation, I did not focus my eyes on the real source of light, but projected my vision right across the room. When one is tired one's eyes tend naturally to roll upward. If there is nothing on which to focus vision, there is no awareness of the movement of the eyeballs. My eyes had rolled upward and, therefore, the retinal image had crossed the retina in the reverse direction, giving me the false perception of a light moving from above downward in relation to my body. The moment I sat up, I became through proprioceptive stimuli oriented for the room and its furniture. The light then took up its appropriate position relative to the bed and I was able to focus my vision on it, whereupon, of course, I saw the figures as figures and no longer simply as a diffuse light.

If a background be indefinite, or it be wilfully disregarded, analogous reactions may take place. This was shewn well with Bartlett's Blot Experiments.[1] Truly amorphous ink blots were presented to his subjects, who were instructed to see what they looked like. There being nothing to be perceived that fitted in accurately with previous experience, there was a wide variation in interpretation and his subjects indulged in many free associations. For instance, one subject gave this account of what he saw. "Girl leaning over a fence or bridge. Hat falls off. Cape blows off.

[1] *Loc. cit.*

Scarf flies up like a flag. She falls, screaming." These free associations tend to arouse memories. One subject saw the suggestion
of a crown in one of the blots, and described his experience in
these words. "I seemed to be back in the Tower of London,
looking at the Crown Jewels. I could see the bars in front of them,
and the men guarding them. I didn't see myself there, but I felt
as if I was there. It was Sunday afternoon. You seem to feel
differently on Sundays somehow, and I felt like that." In some
subjects, an affective reaction came first and then memories explaining this affect. One described the scene of reading a book
about a pansy—a pansy being the interpretation of the blot.
"This subject had," he said, "distinct visual imagery throughout
but never of himself. He came into the scene through having
what he called 'the feel of' an experience. This was common
in other cases also, particularly when what was recalled had
occurred long before. For blot S., for instance, one of the 'reminiscent' subjects wrote 'feel shuddery—a conglomeration of
slimy snails'. Then she said that many years before at a boarding
house at the seaside she had suffered a shock on finding a snail
crawling on a bread plate. The feeling she had then was revived
when she saw this blot, and became so strong that she had to turn
away in disgust. Another subject was reminded by one of the
blots of an operation for cancer that he had seen performed long
before. He described how he had gone into an anatomical class
room not knowing what was the subject of demonstration. The
sudden shock he had then was revived at the sight of the blot.
    "...in all these cases it appeared that the first glance reinstated
a more or less general situation, marked by a particular feel. Then
specific details were developed".
    These phenomena are explicable on the theory of affect exposed
in my book on Emotion. According to this theory, affect is the
effect in consciousness of a flux of image functions that is proceeding co-consciously. In these blot experiments consciousness
had insufficient material to work with; hence it was not crowded
with a flood of images, activated by environmental stimuli, but was
affected rather by the internal flux. We shall have occasion to
consider this kind of process again in the next chapter.
    False perceptions (illusions) illustrate the mechanism of true
perception when they are closely examined. It is then seen that
the falsity of the perception rests on a relative dominance of an

internal flux over the images aroused by the environmental background. This may be the product of a relative strength of the internal processes which intrude themselves on consciousness (the psychopathic type), or of a weakness of the environmental control due to the external stimulus not being in the focus of awareness. In this latter case, the illusion persists until consciousness is directed specifically to that which has been falsely perceived. In most cases, of course, both factors are combined. Professor Bleuler tells the story on himself of seeing his name quoted in a scientific work, the pages of which he was turning over rapidly. He stopped to see what the author had to say and discovered that what had caught his eye was really the word "Blutkoerperchen". We can all confess to similar illusions. I was once reading of some trance-like states in soldiers. The thought came to my mind that the author would have known more about this subject had he read a book by Hoch on Stupors, which I had edited. About five minutes later, while reading a line about one inch from the bottom of the page, my eye was distracted by seeing the name "Hoch" in the last line. When I looked to verify this, what I discovered was:

"it, *H*e may say that, when. . .
essence of su*ch* intention. . . ."

These examples illustrate coerced attention, of course, as well as they do the mechanism of perception. Examples of a more psychopathological nature demonstrate the same principles. One of my patients, for instance, was troubled one day by hearing her companions call out her name "Miss J.". Under subsequent hypnosis, she said that she was thinking of her mother and that the words she heard were "Mrs J.". In all probability, her companions were not calling out at all, so that the phenomenon was essentially an hallucination; but what is interesting about this example is that, when the co-conscious idea came into consciousness, it was rationalized by being made into "Miss". In all cases, we can look on the action of consciousness as a kind of rationalization, no matter whether the adjustment to reality is made with something external or with the subject's notion of what is reasonable, and therefore "real". When this process *is* rational, an accurate perception results.

This view as to the nature of perception is not new. Taine[1] says "The external perception is an internal dream which proves

<hr/>

[1] *Loc. cit.* p. 224.

to be in harmony with external things; and, instead of calling hallucination a false external perception, we must call external perception a *true hallucination*". In comparing the experiences of the abnormal person with hallucinations with those of the normal person, he writes: "...in one case, there are objects and external events, independent of ourselves and real, proved by the ulterior experience of the other senses and by the concurring testimony of other observers, which correspond to our phantoms; while, in his case there is no such correspondence".

Dawes Hicks,[1] in discussing this, asks why an "internal phantom" should appear as an external object at all. Taine has already given his answer, when discussing images, and has given it in much the same terms as I am now using, except that he does not allege that the discrimination between image and perception is a specific function of consciousness:[2]

"The ordinary image then is not a simple, but a double fact. It is a spontaneous consecutive sensation, which, by conflicting with another sensation, primitive and not spontaneous, undergoes lessening, restriction, and correction. It comprises two momentary stages, a first in which it seems localized and external, and a second in which this externality and situation are lost. It is the result of a struggle; its tendency to appear external is opposed and overcome by the stronger and contradictory tendency of the sensation occasioned at the same moment by the action of the nerve. Under this effort it grows weak and thin, it is reduced to a shadow; we call it an image, phantasm, or appearance, and, however vivid or clear it may be, the conjunction of this negation is sufficient to deprive it of its substance; to dislodge it from its apparent position, and to distinguish it from the true sensation."

[1] "On the Nature of Images", *Brit. Jour. Psychol.* vol. xv, part 2.
[2] *Loc. cit.* p. 52.

CHAPTER X

MEANING

WE have seen that perception involves the operation of subsidiary reactions that are set up by the "background" of the object perceived. This background qualifies and controls the reaction to the particular object. Every perception has, therefore, a setting that is an integral part of it. The attendant reactions are, however, merely orienting factors, the central reaction remains more or less constant; that is, in a large series of settings, the principal reaction will remain the same. Perception is, accordingly, *generic*, it calls for a type of reaction which betrays the significance of the object for the organism. We might then say this is the meaning of the object. But in so doing, we should merely be importing into the phenomenon an introspective kind of judgment that would add nothing to the understanding of it. I will, therefore, not use "meaning" to describe reactions that are generic for objects. This is merely meaning in the definition, dictionary, sense.

On the other hand, under certain circumstances, the reaction to a given object may not be generic; it may, indeed, be a reaction typically performed in the presence of another stimulus. It may seem objectively as if the thing were perceived as something quite other than what it is. For example, my ordinary perception of a screw-driver is of a tool the purpose of which is to insert or remove screws, made of certain materials and having certain shape, and so on. This is the dictionary kind of meaning. But I may use it, stuck under a door, to keep the door from slamming. I am using it as a wedge. A behaviouristic onlooker might argue that I perceive it as a wedge, but of course I know it is a screw-driver all the time: that is, subjectively my perception is accurate. I should explain my behaviour by saying that I was using the screw-driver as if it were a wedge. In a certain situation, the meaning of screw-driver has changed for me. The screw-driver under the door no longer has the meaning of screw-drivers in general, that is the

dictionary meaning; it has acquired a *specific* meaning. This latter
is the *psychological meaning*, and exists only when it is different
from the dictionary meaning.

It would appear that it is the setting of the object which determines psychological meaning; in other words, the associated reactions are not serving to orient the central reaction but determine
its very nature, while the object itself is determining the orientation. Naturally, all gradations exist in this shifting of qualifying
or of orientation from object to background or *vice versa*. Whenever there is any specificity of reaction to the setting we can say
that some meaning is appearing. The lower animals shew relatively
little of this, for they have rather a series, large or small, of set
generic perceptions for given objects in a series of varying backgrounds. It would seem, however, that the general environment
may at times determine the nature of the reaction, which has no
relationship whatever to the nature of the immediate stimulus.
This appears, for instance, when there is wide irradiation of conditioned reflexes, such as was discussed in the last chapter. If the
reaction of salivation has been conditioned with a tactile stimulus,
and irradiation is so extensive as to allow an auditory stimulus to
provoke salivation, we are probably forced to conclude that in this
case the sound has merely liberated a response that is conditioned
with the total environment. We must remember that the dog is
in a situation that remains quite unchanged except for variations
in the specific stimuli administered to him. These stimuli belong
to two classes. One is feeding, which excites the inborn reflex of
salivation, and the other is made up of tactile, auditory, etc. stimuli,
which are artificially associated with feeding. No experiment
could be framed in which the animal would be exposed to these
two groups of sensory experience exclusively. He is brought into
a special room, special apparatus is attached to his limbs or his
mouth, and then the experiment begins. The room, the apparatus,
and so on, provide a sensory background which must tend to be
conditioned with feeding and salivation in much the same way as
are the specific conditioned stimuli. This means that the animal
is on the *qui vive* for food. When a strange auditory stimulus
appears, the reaction of salivation, which the background has
activated as liminal images, fires off, because the sound has
excited the animal sufficiently to liberate a reaction which was
potentially present. The meaning of the sound is derived from

the setting of the experiment and not from the nature of the sound itself.

This is, of course, a non-adaptive kind of meaning, because it produces illusion rather than true adaptation to the environment; but, with the utilization of substitutes, there is a beginning of meaning as an adaptive advance on pure perception. The extreme development of psychological meaning appears with the use of symbols where a reaction, oriented to a given object, may bear no relation whatever to the generic qualities of the object. A dog observing a human lover kiss a letter and put it next his heart would probably judge the man to be insane—if the dog were capable of such judgment.

Some excellent examples of totally different reactions to the same object under different circumstances are given in Koehler's book. He describes how chimpanzees frequently smear their bodies, using their hands and applying their own faeces or those of the other apes. This is apparently a practice followed for its own sake: it amuses them, as we would say. But, if they step accidentally on any faeces, they will take an early opportunity of wiping it off with paper, twigs, etc. The same cleansing is done of other accidental foreign matter, including blood, that gets on to the surface of the body; it is always removed with "wipes" of some sort. In the latter cases the meaning of faeces or other foreign matter is "dirt". The same material may mean something else when it is voluntarily applied, and, for what this meaning may be, we had best apply to the psycho-analysts. Another example shews meaning intruded so as to produce stupidity. One of the apes having learned to use a box in order to secure fruit seemed to be totally unable to recognize it as a possible implement if another ape were sitting on it. As soon as the companion would get off, the box could be used.

The study of meaning is, then, a study of associated reactions. The specificity of meaning may come from reactions set up by peculiarities of the environment, or from reactions peculiar to the personality. These latter interest us most and they are best studied where distortion from the dictionary meaning is most glaring, as occurs in psychopathological material. For example, one anxious and depressed patient having heard the word "lobster" spoken, asserted that this signified that he was going to be boiled alive. This patient had a pathological interest in violent death which, we presume, determined the peculiar free associations this word aroused. A normal individual would associate with "lobster" something to eat, restaurant, etc., which would shew little psychological meaning. On the other hand, an individual with a specialized interest might associate to the words Homarus, Arthropoda, etc. One might perhaps say that some psychological meaning was being intruded here as a result of the scientific interest; but this is still only determining a choice well within the range of dictionary meanings. The associations of the patient, however, were probably somewhat on this order: lobster, something to eat, method of preparing for table, violent death, I am to be killed, "lobster" is a veiled threat. The latter two associations are purely personal and absolutely unpredictable from any common knowledge of lobsters or of types of interest in lobsters.

Since these associations are unpredictable, the meaning must rest on the associations taking an unusual and new direction—at least for the first time a new meaning appears. Normally, a given stimulus sets up a train of reactions conditioned with it. In the instance we have just considered, however, death or the threat of death was never associated with "lobster" in actual experience. It must, therefore, have been the product of the combining tendency. This latter appears only in the highest animals and consequently we should not expect to find meaning of personality origin occurring except in man or occasionally perhaps in anthropoids or unusually intelligent dogs, etc. When an unusual association of patterns has been achieved by combination, the direction which the flux of image functions takes is a function of interest and, indeed, we may say that it is one of the indications of interest.

The determination of meaning by special associations is sometimes shewn nicely, and in an almost experimental way, in abnormal mental states produced by physical damage to the brain which interferes with certain kinds of association. I shall select only one example of this, a case of war injury resulting in concussion. It should be remembered that with concussion of the brain there is as a rule "retro-active amnesia", that is, after recovery of consciousness, there is not only a forgetting of the injury itself but also of the events immediately preceding it. The patient was a young American soldier whose chief complaint was of depression consequent on a deep conviction of guilt. He said he had "killed an American officer". When asked for details of this crime, all he could recall was shooting somebody in the uniform of an American officer. Some days later, the amnesia had very largely cleared up, as is quite common in such cases. Coincidently his depression lifted, because he remembered the exact nature of the incident that had been troubling him. His story was a dramatic one. It was in the last few days of the war, when the advance was so rapid that the lines were extended and disorganized. None of the soldiers and few of the junior officers knew exactly where they were, and some small units pushed forward into unknown territory. The patient having a slight headache reported this to his commanding officer, who told him to go to the battalion dressing station and get some medicine. On his way to the point, where he thought the dressing station was, he was met by a man in the uniform of an American officer who began to question him as to the names of the American units in the local operations. Recalling an instruction he had received to answer no such questions, he refused all information; whereupon his interlocutor drew a revolver and ordered the man to accompany him. After walking a couple of hundred yards to a clump of trees, they were joined by two German privates. The American was disarmed and left under guard of one of the privates. A few minutes later, observing that the guard was inattentive, the patient sprang suddenly at him, seized his trench knife and stabbed him. At this point observing the "American officer" returning, he took his late guard's pistol and shot him and then began running in the direction which he took to be "home". Shells began to fall around him and that was all he could remember. Here we have in two phases exactly the same memory, namely that of shooting a man in the uniform of an American officer. The meanings of this incident were diametrically opposed when they were manufactured by associations made up from the patient's general experience or from a specific bit of experience. When the meaning was of the general or dictionary type, guilt and depression were a natural response. When the meaning was derived from the peculiarity of an actual situation, the emotional reaction was of a different nature.

In this case a cure came about spontaneously by the emergence of a memory which changed the meaning. Effective psychotherapy often or always rests on producing a change in meanings. This is the method of psycho-analysis in effect, but is the very essence of the therapeutic theory of Morton Prince, when he endeavours to change the "settings" of unconscious complexes. (The theory of meaning which I am now putting forward is, I believe, in complete harmony with that of Morton Prince although elaborated independently.) We may take, as an example, Prince's famous "Church bells phobia" case. His patient suffered from a peculiar mixture of painful emotional reactions which she associated with Church towers. Investigation shewed first of all that it was the ringing of bells in the towers that excited the unpleasant affect. Through automatic writing the story was revealed of the patient's praying for the recovery of her mother, who was undergoing a serious operation, at the time some neighbouring Church bells were pealing. Subsequent to this incident, either the sound of bells or the sight of a Church tower re-awakened the harrowing affective state that characterized the original occasion. The mere recovery of this memory produced no cure whatever. This was brought about only when an examination was made of the total setting of the original incident. It appeared that the patient had blamed herself for her mother's death, because it took place on a trip that the patient believed had been undertaken by the mother for the patient's sake. It was not difficult, however, to shew that in all probability the mother's pleasure had more to do with the trip than the daughter's. As soon as the patient saw this, the setting—the meaning—of the whole situation was changed and with this the symptom disappeared.

When dealing with psychopathological material, it often seems as if the same object or idea had two meanings for the patient, one a conscious and another unconscious one, owing to there being quite different series of associations consciously and unconsciously to the same stimulus. To avoid confusion, it may be well to have a separate term for this and so, when an object has an unconscious setting different from the conscious meaning, I shall call the former its "significance", reserving "meaning" for conscious qualification. Unconscious significance may be objectively manifest although it is opposed to conscious meaning. When this is so, the former is betrayed by the behaviour of the patient.

Meaning is an expression of interest. Interest, as we have seen, is largely unconscious in its operation and, therefore, meaning must rest frequently on mental processes that are not exposed to the consciousness of the subject. This kind of meaning then appears as an affect attached to the object. Symbols, which bulk so largely in the mental life of human beings, fall into this class, the special meaning which they enjoy being derived almost entirely from the emotional reaction which they engender. There are, then, three ways in which meaning may be exhibited: (1) Behaviour, (2) Affect, (3) Conscious knowledge of the associated patterns. It is probably from this last that abstract thought is developed, as we shall see later.

Recognition is a simple kind of meaning which we must next discuss, and in connection therewith we shall see more of the way in which the attendant associations work.

CHAPTER XI

RECOGNITION

IN studying recognition, we are of course invading the territory of memory: in fact introspectively known memory can be divided for purposes of discussion into recognition and voluntary recall. Recognition is knowing a thing again, that is, it is a cognitive and, therefore, introspective process. However, we are accustomed also to use the term objectively as, for example, when we say that a dog recognizes his master. When one begins to analyse this situation, it seems that we speak of recognition only when the dog, confronted suddenly with his master, goes through behaviour specific for the master and accompanies this by emotional display. We arrive at this conclusion on realizing that we speak of the dog knowing the road home or knowing various objects and people, but that in ordinary speech we confine the term recognition to the more dramatic exhibitions of knowledge. This suggests that there is more in recognition than a mere repetition of generic responses. Proof of this appears in abnormal human states, where there may be a repetition of the generic response without any subjective awareness thereof, and this is associated with revolutionary mental disturbance, including a total absence of recognition, as we shall see.

Katzaroff[1], on the basis of careful experiments, concludes that in recognition there is first an affective reaction, a feeling of familiarity attached to the object of perception, which is immediate and direct; this is followed by an activation of images and memories, more or less specific, which justify or moderate the original feeling of familiarity. The affect is the essential kernel, the memory of the antecedent experience a rationalization. He thinks that the confusion in various accounts of recognition, given by different psychologists, is due to the stress on, or exclusive study of, the second element by practically all authors.

[1] "Contribution à l'Étude de la Récognition", *Archives de Psychologie*, vol. XI, p. 1.

There are two arguments which may be used to justify this view. The first is that we know of the feeling of familiarity existing as a specific and almost isolated affect. This occurs in the peculiar mental state, often spoken of by the layman as "having been there before", and most generally referred to by psychologists as "*déjà vu*". In this phenomenon, the subject is harrowed by a feeling of familiarity attaching to some bit of cognitive experience without being able to recall the antecedent experience of which the present one seems to be an identical reproduction.[1] The second argument is that a mere recall of an antecedent experience, which is practically identical with a present perception, does not produce recognition— if one is using that term with any nicety. For instance, if I am resuming a lecture, it is necessary for me to recall the situation at the close of the previous lecture, but I do not recognize the class; it seems merely familiar to me. This memory is by itself merely voluntary recall. Three problems now emerge: (1) the nature of the situation calling forth a true recognition; (2) the nature of the affect; (3) the nature of the mental processes underlying the affect.

The first is not difficult of discovery. If I meet one of my class in London I recognize him; if I see the same man in my lecture room in Cambridge I do not recognize him, although I know he is there. In these two cases there is a difference of setting: when recognition takes place, the familiar is seen in an unfamiliar place, it is a case of coerced attention. In the lecture room the automatic orientation patterns include the faces of the members of the class; the total situation and every element in it is familiar because habitual, there being nothing striking about it, no feeling of familiarity is engendered. But, when the sight of a face sets up patterns not part of a contemporary orientation, there is a feeling of familiarity. When I meet one of my class in London a familiar object appears in a new setting. A new meaning appears and with this is associated recognition.

The second problem is not so simple. Claparède[2] reduces the affect to a feeling of *me-ness* (moïté) associated with the perception or idea. The recurrence of an idea or reaction without this me-ness, he says, is not recognized. In proof of this, he cites the results he obtained in some post-hypnotic experiments and similar phenomena observed in patients suffering from the Korsakoff syndrome

---

[1] For a discussion of this subject see my *Psychology of Emotion*, chap. XLIII.
[2] "Récognition et Moïté", *Archives de Psychologie*, vol. XI, p. 79.

of symptoms. In both these conditions there may be an accurate reproduction of a reaction with a total absence of the feeling of me-ness and, therefore, complete ignorance of there being any repetition of the experience.

Claparède hypnotized several subjects and then taught them a new and arbitrary set of names for digits. On being awakened, the subjects had no memory whatever of having been taught the new signs, and yet could repeat them when given the digits as stimuli. Sometimes the new names appeared as actual hallucinations. In no case was the subject able to account for the queer syllables that came into his mind when a given number was presented to him.

In the Korsakoff syndrome there may be a similar correct repetition of response without conscious memory of the origin of the association. The Korsakoff syndrome is a peculiar form of mental disease resulting from a variety of physical injuries to the brain, but most commonly as a complication of multiple neuritis following on chronic alcohol poisoning. The condition as a rule begins with a delirium in which the patient imagines himself to be engaged in his customary occupation, he is driving his horses or whatever it may be. When this delirium passes off he is found to have a curious memory defect: although possessed of a tolerably complete memory of events prior to the onset of his illness, he can remember nothing that has occurred since then. He will describe the place where he is as a church, a factory, or what not, say the doctor is his employer or a priest, and, so far as direct answers to questions are concerned, would seem to be completely disoriented for time, place and persons. When his capacity is gone into with careful tests, it is found that this disorientation results from the fact that he can remember nothing for more than a minute or so. This is the customary description of a Korsakoff patient. Claparède, however, noticed that the behaviour of these patients was much more adequate to the real situation than this account would lead one to expect. Although admitting no knowledge of their surroundings, the patients do behave as if they were in a hospital. They will take orders from the doctors and nurses. They know where their beds are, where the dining room is, or the way to the lavatories. That is, when occasion arises they behave as if they knew these things, although, were they questioned at the moment, they could not account accurately for their behaviour. Such observations led Claparède to experiment with the capacity of these patients to reproduce certain acquired responses on a stimulus and response basis. Some quotations will illustrate this.

"If one tells her a little story, if one reads her different items of news from a paper, three minutes afterwards she remembers nothing, not even the fact that one has read her something; one succeeds, however, by certain questions, in resuscitating by a kind of reflex certain details in these items.... But when these details have recurred in consciousness, she does not recognize them as memories, she thinks that something 'has crossed her mind' by chance, she 'has an idea without knowing why', it is a product of her imagination at the moment, or even a result of her reflection."

Katzaroff quotes some of these examples: "He (Claparède) succeeded ...in getting reproduced in a Korsakoff patient certain words he had spoken to her before: the patient repeated the words but without re-cognizing that they were memories, she did not recognize them at all. So Claparède read to her one day an anecdote about a woman of 64 years who took her flock out to pasture and was bitten by a snake. The next day he asked the patient to tell him what he had read to her the day before. This she was unable to do, for she did not even remember that a story had been read to her. M. Claparède then pressed her to speak, trying to evoke automatic memories; he demanded imperatively that she should tell him the age of this woman (in the story): the patient then asked, 'Was not this woman 64 years old?' But she added as well that this was an idea that 'came into her head' that she might 'just as well have said something else'....If one shews a picture to the above patient, she fails to recognize it again in as short a time as 10 to 15 seconds. However, if one asks her next to draw anything she wants, she succeeds in reproducing what is indubitably the figure she has been previously shewn and of which she has retained no conscious memory."

Claparède adds another striking example of a repeated but unrecog-nized reaction. "...I tried the following experiment...to see if she would better retain an intense impression that set affectivity into play. I pricked her hand forcibly with a pin hidden between my fingers. This little pain was as quickly forgotten as indifferent perceptions and, shortly after the pricking, she remembered no more of it. However, when I moved my hand near hers again, she pulled her hand back in a reflex way and without knowing why. If, in fact, I demanded the reason for the withdrawal of her hand, she answered in a flurried way, 'Isn't it allowable to withdraw one's hand?'...If I insisted, she would say to me, 'Perhaps there is a pin hidden in your hand'. To my question 'What can make you suspect that I would like to prick you', she would take up her refrain, 'It is an idea which came into my head', or some-times she would try to justify herself with, 'Sometimes pins are hidden in hands'. But she never recognized this idea of pricking as a memory".

8-2

The feeling of me-ness is, according to Claparède, something that has its original appearance with careful examination or scrutiny of anything new: the experience is then stamped as something that is *mine*. (This gives it meaning, I should say.) When recognition occurs this feeling is re-awakened with the memory, according to Claparède. It would seem, however, that this formula is a little incomplete, for it is plain that the feeling of me-ness is more than a mere feeling that the memory is my own mental process. It has a retrospective slant: it is a feeling of me-ness associated with the memory, when the memory is known to be a memory. In other words, it refers to a me-ness in the past. Also it carries with it a mild or strong compulsion to activate the memory, expanding its detail. If I see a face, feel it to be familiar and cannot get the name or other identification at once, I am uncomfortable, until I succeed in arousing these further data. Me-ness refers, therefore, to the past and includes an urge to recall the original situation. This compulsive element may become painful, as in *déjà vu*, and then is apt to carry with it a colouring of perplexity.

The third problem is the discovery of the mental processes underlying this peculiar affect. In studying *déjà vu*, it is found that the affect is due to the arousal of the memory of something (as co-conscious images?) similar in nature to the immediate exciting stimulus; this memory does not penetrate into consciousness. Some kind of inhibition keeps it out, the affect only appearing in consciousness, and the latter persists so long as the deadlock lasts. Two factors are involved: one is the pertinacity of the co-conscious processes (dominance of the interest represented) and the other is the strength of the repression. Normally, no strong repression is present, the affect is then of extremely short duration and may pass unnoticed, unless remarked by an eager introspection. It is, therefore, the abnormal state which provides the better material for investigation. A study of this seems to indicate that the intensity of affect corresponds to a dominance of a co-consciously operating interest. We do not find *déjà vu* with a failure to recall simple experience unconnected with the emotional life of the subject, and so we conclude that the affect comes more from the unconscious processes than from the conscious perception that has precipitated the total reaction. The haunting feeling of familiarity is the conscious expression of pertinacious co-conscious images of something similar; the compulsion to recall the earlier experience—like all compulsions—is the unconscious interest striving for expression, although blocked by repression. The latter element is important: the sight of a vaguely familiar face does not produce true *déjà vu* unless it is that of someone emotionally important to the subject, or of a person resembling such an one. If the person seen or the person co-consciously recalled does not bulk largely in the instinctive life of the subject, he passes on and thinks no more about it.

The feeling of familiarity is central to the process of recognition, but is not recognition itself. Were it so, recognition would never go further than the mere feeling of familiarity and be no more adaptive than is *déjà vu*. It is merely a surface and subjective manifestation of the operation of processes that go on to recognition. When the co-consciously activated processes are not inhibited, and are strong enough to maintain attention, they come into consciousness. There then occurs the final stage in recognition which is an intellectual judgment of identity. Here there are three possibilities: correct judgment, false judgment (false recognition), or judgment of dissimilarity. Examples of these three are "Yes, that is Smith, whom I met at so and so": or "That is Jones, my old friend": or "That man reminds me of Jones, but he is really a stranger". Any one of these judgments puts an end to the affect and to the whole process. False recognition occurs when a dominance of interest overwhelms conscious judgment and so produces an illusion. This is well illustrated in the constant mis-identifications of those about them on the part of patients in manic excitement; the important actors in the patient's trend are impersonated, as it were, by fellow-patients and hospital attendants.

This theory assumes that unconscious processes anticipate conscious ones, although the time interval may be so short as to make the two seem simultaneous to casual introspection. In my book on Emotion I have reviewed a considerable amount of evidence for this claim derived particularly from the study of dreams and the experimental observations of Morton Prince. This is, of course, material of a psychopathological order. But if one be on the look out for it, one may detect occasionally and under peculiar circumstances examples of co-conscious processes anticipating conscious reactions in normal life. I may quote one example of this:[1]

[1] *Psychology of Emotion*, p. 556.

...."A man passed me on a bicycle, who looked familiar. A quick scrutiny of his face convinced me that I did not really know him, but he reminded me of someone else. After several seconds I succeeded in summoning the memory of this other man. It was a friend S., whom I had not seen for a long time and was then on the other side of the Atlantic. Coincidentally with the resuscitation of this memory, so far as I could tell, I saw a Cambridge undergraduate in cap and gown but carrying a golf bag slung over his shoulder. An incongruous combination! He was about fifty feet distant from me and at an angle of about thirty degrees from the axis of my eyes. At once I turned my eyes to get the spectacle in the centre of vision and as soon as I had done so, the golf bag disappeared.although the undergraduate, cap and gown were there all right. The hallucination cannot have lasted more than a fraction of a second, although it was distinct and definite. I actually could describe the golf bag in detail. It took very little longer for me to discover the origin of the hallucination. I am very fond of golf and I played it frequently with S.

This is a good example of one of the functions of co-conscious images. Some detail of the bicyclist's face (probably his moustache) evoked an image of my friend S., that was latent in the unconscious. It became conscious and exhibited itself at first only in a feeling of familiarity. The next step should have been the immediate translation of the image 'S.' into the conscious thought 'S.'. But I was tired. Therefore, it was easier to allow a more primitive type of thinking, a flux of images, to proceed co-consciously than to have the process elaborated from image to conscious thought. An habitual interest— golf—implies a low threshold for stimulation of the image processes connected with it. So, co-consciously, I associated from S. to golf. This was a 'dream' and like a dream, entered consciousness only as one fragment that was rationalized at once by attaching it to something in the environment. But this something was not in the centre of vision and hence not in the focus of awareness. The moment I got it there, consciousness abolished the rationalization and turned the hallucination into an image."

Since the whole efficiency of consciousness rests on the speed of its action, it is natural that such observations as the above should be very rarely possible. On the other hand, it is not difficult artificially to introduce a disturbance in the relationship between conscious and unconscious mental processes, roughly analogous to what takes place in dreaming. A number of drugs may accomplish this. For instance, mescalin seems to bring into consciousness processes normally co-conscious. When this occurs, the latter appear preponderantly in image form (as with Morton Prince's hypnotic material) and so hallucinations result, although there may be insight as to the abnormal character of these sensory

presentations. Such an alteration in thinking is, of course, revolutionary and brings, therefore, other changes in its train. When
these images, produced under the influence of mescalin, are available in introspection the parallelling of thinking in terms of
images and of abstractions may be noted. The following example[1]
illustrates this:

"The subject K. sees coloured lines and points as well as fine red
and white flakes that move here and there in the visual field. He is
ordered to imagine them rotating. A disc of concentric circles appears
that remain still; if the subject so wills, they rotate. Command: 'Imagine
a rotation from the front to the left and from the back to the right'. K.
delays with his answer because he does not understand the order at
once. Suddenly he describes an hallucinated apparent movement,
that corresponds to the directions exactly, without his having been clear
about them until now. It is only from the hallucinated movement that
he recognizes this to be an execution of the imagination demanded."

This analysis of recognition involves voluntary recall as part of
the recognition process. In fact, it could be said that recognition
is a feeling of familiarity which stimulates, and leads over into,
voluntary recall, with a final step of comparison of the images
thus evoked with the perception at hand. Our consideration of
recognition cannot, then, be regarded as complete until we have
analysed voluntary recall, which will be attempted in the next
chapter. Assuming, however, the existence of voluntary recall as
a separable step in the total process, the above formula may stand
as a description of what is involved in recognition.

A theory that does not account equally well for normal and
abnormal phenomena is psychologically incompetent. We must,
therefore, examine further the failure of recognition and voluntary
recall in the Korsakoff syndrome and in the post hypnotic state,
which Claparède sums up as absence of me-ness. In both these
conditions the immediate perception activates patterns that bring
appropriate responses into consciousness. What is further lacking?
Let us consider the Korsakoff syndrome first.

I think there can be no doubt as to the facts which Claparède
reports, for (in complete ignorance at the time of his work) I made
quite similar observations on these patients. Let us analyse the
Korsakoff picture in the terms I have been using in this book.
Beginning with the most complicated mental processes, we find

---

[1] Guttmann, "Medikamentöse Spaltung der Persönlichkeit", *Monatsschr. f.
Psychiatrie u. Neurologie*, Bd. LVI, H. 2/3, S. 170.

that consciousness is intact, or relatively so, except during the delirious stage. This is shewn by the fact that the patient can use images well (accurate solution of form board problems, picture completion tests, etc.); he has too a capacity to reason (perfect accomplishment of watch tests). The combining capacity seems to be intact: in fact, it works if anything overtime, resulting in amusing rationalizations that are technically known as fabrications. For instance, one of my patients whose name was Kavanaugh when asked to spell his name gave, very carelessly, Ka - va - na - gh. When the absence of the u was pointed out to him, he remarked that the doctor he saw two weeks ago told him to leave out the u as it would save time. Again, when unable to give details of an interview with the doctor half an hour before, he said he had been unwilling to keep him long, the doctor was a busy man with a large family, and so on. The Korsakoff patient tends constantly to compensate for his memory defect with such fabrications, all of which involve use of the combining capacity. As to the utilization of substitutes I have made no specific tests, but I think it safe to presume that this capacity is present, judging from the normality of the patient's behaviour. Registration of new impressions is practically normal. For example, the patient can repeat a string of digits or a string of words or imitate a series of movements with perfect accuracy up to that point where the length of time involved in the repetition exceeds the interval during which his memory can operate. He has, then, no incapacity of responding to new stimuli. There remains to be considered his capacity for conditioning new reactions.

There can be no doubt that this capacity is present. Like Claparède I was struck by the inconsistency between the behaviour and the conscious memory of these patients. As I have said, they know their way about the wards, they ask questions of the right people, they will even inadvertently call the physician "doctor", although a moment later fabricating a different profession for him. In a word, they behave as if they knew they were in hospital. I have made a number of tests of their capacity to repeat associations already present. When tested, at intervals of days, with the same word association tests, they will give an unusually high percentage of the same responses and, moreover, betray emotional disturbance with precisely the same complex indicators. This, of course, is what one would expect, considering the normality of their behaviour and their correct use of objects: if the series of associations, on which their responses were based while well, had been disturbed, they would have become totally incompetent. Their capacity to retain new associations apart from their obvious incapacity voluntarily to recall them, I discovered in a series of "guessing" experiments. I would give to the patient my full name and address. Within a few minutes this was totally "forgotten". Later on, I would present the patient with a list of ten Christian names, another of ten surnames, another of street numbers, and another of street names. From these he would be asked to guess which one was mine. To my surprise, the guesses were nearly as accurate as would be the conscious memory for such data of normal subjects. But the response remained to the subject a sheer guess, it was associated with no feeling of me-ness; on no occasion did the patient think that he had the slightest reason for picking one name rather than another from the list. We see, then, that, although the patient may have conditioned these responses in part, the reactions cannot be elicited without the presence as a stimulus of the element which ought to be completely imaged, were the process of conditioning complete. In other words, the correct responses are represented only as liminal images.

Plainly, the defect of the Korsakoff patient, when analysed out into terms of these different processes, is not absolute but relative. The problem then is to discover which one of these capacities is weakest and, through its weakness, gives rise to an almost total failure of recognition and of voluntary recall. At our suggestion, Wechsler[1] tested the capacity for forming new associations in five patients. He gave two lists of ten paired words each, the first pairs being logical (preformed associates) and the second illogical (new associations).

"Before experiment was begun subject was given the following instructions: The experimenter was going to read to him ten pairs of words. He must listen carefully to these ten pairs, and remember the first word of each pair in connection with the second. After the list of ten pairs had been read through the experimenter would take a little rest and then read the first word of each pair, and he (subject) must give him the second word. If he gave the correct associate the experimenter would say 'that's right' and continue, but if subject did not remember the word, the experimenter would supply it. If he should

[1] "A Study of Retention in Korsakoff Psychosis", *Psychiatric Bulletin of the New York State Hospital*, vol. II, no. 4.

happen to give the wrong word, the experimenter would say 'no' and then give him the right word."

"The Korsakoff cases shewed a marked disturbance in the formation of new associations.

"(a) They were able to reproduce habitually preformed associations almost as readily as normal individuals, but as these became less of an habitual sort the associations were less readily reproduced. This was shewn in the tests on preformed associates.

"(b) Korsakoffs were almost wholly unable to form new associations. This was shewn by the tests on the formation of new associations. Whereas normal individuals could learn to associate ten pairs of un-related words in from three to five trials (median 4 P.E. 1) none of the Korsakoffs was able to get more than two in twenty trials and four of the five Korsakoffs could not get any."

"An analysis of the errors shewed a preponderance of false associa-tions over failure to recall associates, a condition which contrasted very strikingly with that found in normal subjects.

"There was a marked tendency to perseverate any false associations once made. Such false associations were not diminished through cor-rection, but rather increased, at least relatively, with the number of repetitions."

An examination of the errors shews that the "false associations" and "perseverations" were merely a product of the patient's own preformed associations.

Now to interpret these findings. The normal behaviour of the Korsakoff patient is to be ascribed to a substitution of the new stimuli in the patient's preformed patterns, which is accomplished after countless repetitions. That is, he has learned in his normal life to respond to the kind of situation which he meets with in the hospital, and all he has now to do is to modify these patterns slightly, so that appropriate new responses may appear when he is con-fronted with the various slightly new stimuli belonging to the hospital. It is important to note, however, that these new patterns are only exhibited when the appropriate stimuli are actually present, in other words these new patterns are composed of liminal images: were there full-fledged image functions the patient would be conscious of why he was behaving in a correct manner and not be, consciously, disoriented. We can now trace the effect of this weakness in the formation of new associations as it appears in the different stages of the psychosis.

When only preformed associations are in existence, perceptions are merely activated images, that is, there are hallucinations or at best illusions. This gives the first stage of occupation delirium.

As the delirium subsides, some new patterns are being built with links of liminal images. There is now a correct perception for common objects in their new relationships, but there is no perception of unique objects. For example, the identity of the people around is something totally new. So, at this stage, we find misidentification and fabrication, and this stage may persist indefinitely. We have here a "background" for common objects, but no "background" for unique objects or unique experiences. In other words, there is very limited meaning. In the last stage some liminal images have become images, as the reaction to unique elements is more thoroughly conditioned. The presence of true images is shewn by the ability of the patient to perform small acts of primitive planning: he can image the situation of his bed, etc., and so go to it when he wishes. Correct behaviouristic orientation has been achieved and there is no longer fabrication except under duress.

This is the ordinary chronic Korsakoff. Why does improvement not proceed further? It is because, with his limited capacity for building new associations, he has learned the reactions appropriate to objects in their new situations, but only in so far as these situations are unvarying. In a normal person, the correct reaction to a comparatively new situation is learned in one experience of it. That means that a process, taking weeks or months for the patient, is acquired at once. Otherwise intelligent, the Korsakoff has suddenly become as ineducable as a rather stupid dog. (This is the natural tendency with advancing age, and it is interesting that some senile individuals develop the Korsakoff picture, then called presbyophrenia.) With the correct response to a stimulus in a normal human being, the subsidiary reactions set up by the background are conditioned as well. The latter are side-chains, not part of the central reaction. The Korsakoff patient may react properly enough to the background stimuli, but, unless these stimuli are invariably repeated, he cannot build up new patterns combining the accessory with the central reactions. In other words, meanings are for him incapable of reproduction, although he can exhibit them whenever an actual situation calls for a discriminative response. Consider, for instance, the meaning of his physician to the Korsakoff patient. In a series of encounters, the patient behaves with the peculiar deference he has always exhibited towards a doctor. This reaction is then conditioned with the perception of the particular doctor, who now calls forth the habitual "doctor" response. Sight of the physician will be sufficient to produce appropriate, deferential behaviour;—it is interesting that, even when misidentification is at its height, the doctor is never called by the name of one of the patient's own class, he is always dubbed a priest, lawyer, employer, etc. Now, in this series of correct responses, such data as the medical officer's name, his title, or the subject spoken of are not invariably repeated. Hence, the sight of the doctor does not cause his name to spring to the patient's lips, nor even yet his title, for these are subsidiary, unconditioned elements in the behaviour series. Only what is central, unvarying and integral in correct behaviour towards a given individual can be reproduced.

This brings us to a point where we can identify a little more accurately the origin and basis of me-ness. A most important attendant reaction in normal people is conscious awareness of what one is doing, i.e. voluntary attention. As this too is not integral to a correct response, the Korsakoff patient fails to condition this with his behaviour. Consequently, there is no connection remaining after the event between the act and the personality. Retrospectively, although the response may be resuscitated as a mere response, it does not carry with it any association with the personality. It was not done by *me*, it did itself, so to speak. This, of course, is not a phenomenon unknown in normal life. The things we deny ever having done, in the face of ample testimony from honest observers, are acts performed "absent-mindedly", automatically. Automatic behaviour has no me-ness attached to it.

We have seen above that the strength of the feeling of familiarity depends on the range of the co-consciously operating interests. In Korsakoff only simple behaviour patterns are involved as a rule, so very little feeling of familiarity is engendered even in an environment for which specific responses have been learned. It follows, however, from this interpretation of the Korsakoff psychosis, that if a situation had arisen which involved a powerful interest, producing in turn a reaction of which consciousness was an essential link, then this incident might be subsequently recognized and voluntarily recalled. It is a commonplace of animal behaviour studies that reactions are much more easily conditioned when powerful appetites are involved. If an interest were sufficiently powerful, it would not lapse with the cessation of the act but would be apt to cause immediate and repeated rehearsal of the act in fantasy. This might be sufficient to cause an integration of the various elements therein, including the links of personality and consciousness. These conditions are fulfilled when delusions are present (pathological and dominating interests), producing conduct in which affect (a phenomenon of consciousness) is one of the integral stimuli in a train of behaviour.

I shall quote one example of this briefly. The patient had suffered from a stroke in consequence of a syphilitic lesion in his brain. On recovering consciousness he was, for some weeks, so aphasic as to be almost completely unintelligible. When understandable speech returned, it was discovered that he had such a severe retention defect that he could remember nothing for more than fifteen or twenty seconds—that is, so far as tests revealed his memory. But, while still in the delirious phase, he was preoccupied more with delusions than with recollections of his normal life; these delusions were not forgotten! Many of them were concerned with fears for his bodily safety. Reassurance would dispel the delusions, but these reassurances would be forgotten at once, so that in a few minutes the delusions would return in full force, the comforting thoughts could not be conditioned with the patterns making up the pathological interests. On one occasion, while in a panic, he wrote a curious letter to his brother, consisting of one sentence in which all the words were French except one. (He was bilingual.) What he wrote was: "Il faut que to viens me prendre d'ici tout de suite si tu veux me voir alive". This letter he did not forget, in fact a year later he could repeat it word for word, even including the one English word! It is important to note that this striking memory was of an event which occurred in a sequence that included the affect of terror as an integral link. Fear was the stimulus for writing the letter, it was not an accessory reaction. It was a sequence, therefore, in which consciousness was an essential element, hence it was possible for it to be integrated with the personality, to be dowered with me-ness.

Claparède says:[1] "The feeling of me-ness is, so to speak, the link by which a memory-image is bound to the ego, the link by which we maintain it, and thanks to which we can draw it up from the depths of the unconscious. If this link is broken, we lose at the same stroke the possibility of recalling it voluntarily". This

[1] *Loc. cit.* p. 87.

is just my view, except that for "feeling" I would substitute "co-conscious processes that are registered in consciousness as feeling". It seems to me impossible that anyone could study the Korsakoff syndrome and maintain the behaviourist view that consciousness—the phenomenon or the concept—is unessential.

It is, perhaps, unfair to demand of behaviourists a knowledge of the Korsakoff syndrome; but children, whose reactions they observe sedulously, exhibit quite analogous "symptoms". For instance, we can take the report of W. S. Hunter on the youngest child used in his Delayed Reaction experiments, to which I have already referred at considerable length. On p. 59, he makes the statement that F., aged two and a half years, delayed well up to fifty seconds and badly up to one minute, which was her limit for correct delayed reactions. The older children, however, did well up to intervals of more than half an hour, and Hunter notes that with the latter the "purpose to remember" was an important aid. Here he uses a phrase that has a definite meaning for introspection, but seems irrelevant to a psychology, purporting to deal merely with stimulus and response. Other psychologists are prepared to admit that consciousness is not present at birth but develops later, and that when it does appear certain types of behaviour are made possible for the first time.

We would say that F. had not yet acquired voluntary recall. What does Hunter say? (p. 61) "...the child was just reaching the stage where her memory for objects and events had begun to take on a definite form. When brought in from a ride in the park or a visit to a friend, she could very seldom remember the details of the event, indeed not more than half the time could she remember the gross fact of having been somewhere. This occurred even with what were to F. very interesting experiences. Sometimes, it is true, the difficulty lay with the lack of control of language; but this was not always the case. After her playmate had gone for some time, if F. was asked who had been there, not only could she frequently not tell, but at times she was bewildered by the suggestion that anyone had been to see her at all. On the other hand, some cases were noted where F. remembered an event for several days. Phrases, also, that she had heard but once were often spontaneously repeated for the first time several days later". Anyone with a psychological interest, who has observed little children, would confirm the accuracy of this description. The vagaries of their memory are astounding, until it is realized that they have little or no voluntary recall. If a given situation happens to excite the right train of associations, they may produce a memory of something that occurred a full year before. But there is nothing to guide the direction of the associations except their larval interests, so that fantasy is as likely to appear as an accurate memory.

In his experiments, Hunter was—psychiatrically speaking—giving a retention test. The result was like that obtained in Korsakoff patients. In them the clinical picture results from a capacity for conditioning so weak that no association of reactions with consciousness is attained. In little children the association does not occur, partly for the same reason perhaps, but chiefly because there is very little consciousness in existence as yet. The easiest explanation for the change in children's memories as they grow older is the development of a new function called consciousness. On the principle of parsimony—to which the behaviourists are devoted—it ought to be accepted.

There remain to be considered the analogous failures of recognition in the posthypnotic experiments of Claparède. A large variety of studies of hypnotism have revealed conditions there quite like the disturbances produced in Korsakoff by physical agencies. In deep hypnosis the only reactions that seem to be activated are those dictated by the hypnotist. Except when instructed by the hypnotist, the somnambulist remains motionless and anaesthetic. Three results follow relentlessly: (1) the only associations formed are those prescribed; (2) personality as such, therefore, does not enter into the determination of the subject's behaviour (Janet claims that this is a *sine qua non* of suggestion); (3) the personality having no integration with the somnambulism, there is no connection existing, posthypnotically, with the events thereof, so a conscious amnesia results inevitably.

Analysis of recognition leads, then, to the following conclusion: A perception stimulates unconscious interest which in turn activates an image of something similar; this affects consciousness as a feeling of familiarity. This image has been associated with consciousness and the personality, and, hence, may be voluntarily recalled, i.e. brought into consciousness again. A comparison is, then, instituted between the immediate perception and the memory; if they coincide, recognition takes place.

Misunderstandings due to confusion in the use of terms are so common that it may be well to emphasize again the sense in which I am employing the word "recognition". The various "faculties" so overlap and melt into each other, that a loose usage of psychological terms is only natural on the part of the layman. For instance, he tends to use recognition both as perception and memory. As with "meaning", so here I am trying to give to recognition a special connotation, as a peculiar type of memory process. I would make it include all those mental events that have to do with the asking and answering of the question, Where have I had this experience before?

I have analysed recognition into three phases, feeling of familiarity, voluntary recall and judgment of identity. Whether it be right to confine the term only to this syndrome, while denying its pertinence if all three elements are not present, is a matter that is bound to be settled by the taste of individual psychologists and the suitability of this definition for their systems of psychology. I merely insist that there is such a congeries of mental processes as do form a unitary group, and that it does suit my system thus to delimit the term. My justification is that, if all three elements are not present, what I call recognition does not take place.

If there is only a feeling of familiarity, *déjà vu* occurs, which is certainly not normal recognition. If there is no such feeling, there is only a repetition of response, accompanied by an attention which is devoted to the object and not to the historical origin of the behaviour. For example, when I meet a companion that I see daily and meet him under the customary circumstances, I greet him by name as a habit reaction and do not make any of the fuss over it which recognition would involve. If the recall element be automatic, it merges over into the response without any attention being paid to it voluntarily. In this case, the feeling of familiarity is extremely brief and so mild as not to impress a normal introspection. (In fact this mild affect is of the same order as that attaching to all perceptions that feel "real", a general colouring that becomes conspicuous only when it is absent, as in some depressions.) In other words, if the recall is automatic and not voluntary, there is again merely a habit response. It is when the recall does not come spontaneously that voluntary effort is necessary. This means delay, and a consequent enhancement of the affect, on the one hand, with awareness of the memory as such, on the other. The necessity for a judgment of identity is a corollary of the first two elements. Intrinsic to the affect is an urge to bring into consciousness an image identical with what is being perceived. An essential function of consciousness is discrimination of images. The affect originates, as we have seen, in a co-conscious flux of similar images; the only thing that will put an end to this (apart from orientation of the subject to some entirely new object) is the emergence of the images and their acceptance by consciousness.[1] The acceptance is the judgment of identity. If there is no acceptance, consciousness keeps the attention fixed on the object, so that it excites associations to more images, until an appropriate one appears. For instance, I may see a man who excites a feeling of familiarity and may try to evoke data of identification. If he has slanting eyes, images of Chinamen may appear; but the man before me is not a Chinaman. I keep on looking at his face, and images of Europeans I know who have slanting eyes emerge. Finally, the right one comes.

For psychologists, the problem of recognition may be obscured by the intrusion of eager introspection where it would normally never occur; that is to say, the psychologist may scrutinize mental events, whose nature is essentially automatic, that would be performed equally well without the intrusion of consciousness. Recognition, as I use the term, involves introspection, but this is an attention directed internally and coerced by the peculiar affect of familiarity. If, however, attention be voluntarily turned to the processes involved in an otherwise automatic mental event, an artificial kind of recognition may be fabricated. Supposing the psychologist introspects an act of recall that really is spontaneous. To him, the evocation of the memory may seem to be a result of wilful effort, so that it will appear to be an act of voluntary recall. Or, again, he may direct his attention to a judgment of identity and thus dower it with a conative flavour. In either case, he has succeeded in producing a subjective situation very like that he has experienced when he has had a true recognition in my sense of the term. In this, consciousness is more of an onlooker or slave, and neglect of the affective element is, therefore, less likely to occur, for it is what coerces the attention. It is for reasons such as these that I have preferred to base my argument on psychopatho-

---

[1] "Acceptance" is a description not an explanation of the event. For the latter we must wait for the chapter on Inhibition in Part II.

logical evidence, which cannot be wilfully duplicated, using intro-spection only in confirmation.

The claim I have just made, that recognition can be largely manufactured *ad hoc*, follows from the study of attention. What gains attention depends on a threshold established by an inter-action of stimulus and interests. In normal recognition, attention is drawn to the current mental processes by the strength of the affect, on the one hand, and, on the other, by the necessity of gaining data of identification, so that there may be adequate adapta-tion to the immediate situation. Ordinarily, if I pass a familiar face in the street, the strength of the affect (unconscious interest) will determine whether voluntary recall is instituted or persisted in. Or, if I have to speak to the owner of the face, his name would be an advantageous possession. But the adaptation demand may arise from an academic interest in the phenomena of mind: I may ask the question, "Where have I had this experience before?" out of psychological curiosity, and thus manufacture the recognition processes artificially in a situation where the layman would have nothing but a perception. If I want to rationalize a correct re-sponse—if I want to justify a perception—I must resuscitate its background. This effort is part of true recognition. The moment I am forcing the emergence of data to justify a response, I am doing something so like the recovery of data to justify an affect of familiarity, that it may be difficult to discriminate between the two. In normal recognition, consciousness intervenes to solve a problem that is forced upon it. In the artificial type, the problem is created by the personality, by consciousness. The resulting phenomena may be almost identical.

CHAPTER XII

VOLUNTARY RECALL

MEMORY, taken as a repetition of reaction, is merely the activation of a pattern on presentation of the stimulus which corresponds to one of the images that are integrated together to form the pattern. Provided one goes no further than this in considering the phenomena of memory, it is not necessary to take consciousness into account. In fact, memory, in this wide sense, is just another way of saying that the existence of patterns is demonstrable. What particular pattern will be activated—what automatic memory—is determined by appetite or interest. There is no new problem here, for we are merely saying that whenever we encounter a chain of reactions or patterns we are meeting with a series of memories. Free associations are thus a series of automatic memories and psycho-analytic research has shewn how extensive the range of this kind of memory may be. When, on the other hand, we consider the type of memory that normally excites introspection and into which conscious conation enters, two problems arise. These are voluntary recall and judgment as to the validity of the memory evoked. (I do not attempt to discuss validity itself, which is an epistemological or philosophical problem.)

In studying the anomalies of voluntary recall occurring in the Korsakoff syndrome, we have concluded that this process rests on the conditioning of attendant, orienting reactions with a given situation which is to be recalled; and that consciousness, personality, must enter into the complex if there is to be voluntary recall. This complex gives a specific setting for the original perception, that is, it is a meaning. Meanings (as we shall see later) may be integrated into units and can then act as if they were simple images, becoming elements in new, more complicated patterns. A meaning can, therefore, be activated as can an image by the same associational process as in automatic memory. Thus, if I put to myself the question "What did I have for breakfast?", there arise spontaneously the complex "breakfast", and the same complex plus meaning "my breakfast". These associations tell me merely that I have had breakfast because the question automatically brings that association to mind. So long as "my breakfast" remains a unitary complex, I get no further. But meanings, being highly complicated, are unstable. If a meaning be held in consciousness instead of serving as a junction point in passage to a different set of patterns, it breaks up into its parts, that is, when attention is held unwaveringly on the complex itself, the associated reactions of which it is composed and which are perhaps co-consciously activated already, come into consciousness. I then have images of different articles of food, my letters, the newspaper, the time on the clock opposite me, etc.

This process of breaking up of the complex may be illustrated in the visual experiences we have on seeing electric carriage calls, that consist of a mass of electric lights which are illuminated in different patterns to represent different numbers. If one glances at one of these and perceives the lights as a unitary whole, a number is perceived, which is the normal stimulus for another reaction on the part of the beholder. If he be a chauffeur whose number is displayed, he will move to the door of the theatre. If, however, the meaning of the sign be neglected and scrutiny be directed towards its physical composition, it will immediately be analysed out into a number of separate electric lights. These two reactions are analogous to the responses to the questions "Have you had breakfast?" and "What have you had for breakfast?" This is the basic mechanism of voluntary recall: consciousness holds a given stimulus in awareness and this causes an activation of the reactions previously conditioned with it; as these in turn appear in awareness, consciousness criticizes them, rejecting the irrelevant and branding the relevant as valid memory.

The problem is complicated by the fact that in voluntary recall (as in other memories) words are utilized. In the process of human education, words are conditioned both with objects and meanings. A series of images or meanings may then be translated into words and the latter may be the only representations in consciousness of the flux. When this has happened a number of times, the string of words is itself conditioned together, thus forming a verbal pattern. These verbal patterns may then function as mnemonics, and many of our memories are simply verbal patterns. For instance, "the Norman Conquest 1066" is such a verbal pattern with me. In recalling one of these, volition enters in only in so far as the particular pattern is actively sought: the habit of associating certain words together may be so strong that the mention of one will call up the others inevitably. For instance, mention either of Hastings or 1066 will with me cause an instant appearance of the verbal pattern "Battle of Hastings in 1066".

Past experience is then recalled *via* one of two types of patterns —imaginal or verbal. The former is more primitive and fundamental. Since the facility of activation of imaginal patterns is dependent on interest, it follows that interest will determine the memory of remote events. (Remote events are those not linked by immediate association with the present situation.) A corollary of this is important. Our study of attention shewed that the activation of one set of patterns involves the abolition of others. If certain groups of interest be dominant, there will, therefore, be, at the same time, an inhibition of patterns irrelevant to these dominant interests. It follows from this that events experienced, and *ipso facto* establishing new patterns by conditioning, may be actively forgotten. It should be understood, of course, that this active forgetting is not an expression of voluntary effort, but something that takes place outside the range of conscious awareness. It is, indeed, the repression to which so much attention has been directed by psychopathologists, particularly of the psychoanalytic school. This is too obvious a matter to deserve more than mere mention.

When interest, based on an extensive series of patterns that are mostly unconscious, is stimulated, an affect is apt to appear. At least, in so far as interest is operating at any given moment in unconscious reverberations, there is an emotional reaction. Hence, any experience exciting affect is likely to be linked up with interest and, therefore, the more easily recalled—unless the interest be of a pathological order, i.e. foreign to the personality. In the latter case, it will either be actively forgotten or appear as a compulsive symptom. Bartlett[1] noted that pictures exciting affect were the most easily recalled; that is, in my terminology they were built into existing and important patterns.

The next problem is the *judgment of validity*. When any datum is recalled it is either accompanied by a conviction of

---

[1] "The Functions of Images", *Brit. Jour. Psychol.* vol. XI, part 3.

certitude that makes it valid to the subject or this conviction is absent. In the latter case, the subject says "I think it is so and so, but I am not sure". Some examples will make this difference clear. I think that Julius Caesar came to Britain in 55 B.C. But, as I criticize this memory, I am not sure. It might be the date of his assuming the title of emperor or of his death. Considering further, I eliminate the latter possibility, because there comes to my mind the association 45 B.C. in connection with Julius Caesar, but I get no further, and so there is no certitude. On the other hand, that the Battle of Hastings occurred in the year 1066 I am quite certain, although having to admit that I have no proof of this even to myself. When, however, I recall that the late European war began in 1914 and ended in 1918, I am not only certain that my memory is valid but I am convinced that I can prove it. In these three instances, associations appear that affect consciousness differently. In the first, a purely verbal pattern "Julius Caesar 55 B.C." appears; Julius Caesar, not being an event, I know that the association must be between the date and some event in the career of Julius Caesar, but I have no knowledge of which one it was. (On further reflection I recall the real origin of this verbal pattern: it comes from the story of the showman who exhibited a tortoise so ancient that Julius Caesar had carved his name thereon, adding the date 55 B.C. The pattern, in this case, is not associated with any interest that could be labelled "historical" by the most indulgent of critics.) In the second instance, the association is verbal and specific, and so automatic that I am convinced it is right. If it be challenged, however, I have to admit that it is only a verbal pattern, standing quite isolated in consciousness. In the third case, however, I have not only the auditory and visual verbal pattern "World War 1914–1918", but with this are associated innumerable other patterns. If the validity of this memory be challenged, I think of a host of incidents connected with the beginning and the ending of the War, each one of which has a calendar association. In other words, the third memory has extensive meaning which includes temporal factors. The meaning of 1066 is the Conquest which has no time factors in it, because I have forgotten the events immediately preceding and following it, or rather, such few events as I can recall have no dates attached to them.

Under any ordinary circumstances, we do not rehearse all these attendant associations with vivid, conscious awareness thereof. They provide rather a background (like perception) which affects consciousness as a feeling of validity, or as a judgment thereof, if validity is called in question. Certitude depends on the richness of the associations. Hence, a pathological liar, who invents innumerable details as his tale expands, believes his own fabrications.

There are two types of background, meaning of the me-ness kind and a meaning derived from an objective setting. In the first, there are images (of objects or of isolated words), which are valid because they are recognized. This type gives great detail, although it may be haphazard and not particularly adaptive. People with prodigious memories belong as a rule to this type. In the second, we find that data are registered and recalled in virtue of their incorporation into systems that have meaning or, rather, give meaning to the data. These memories are adaptive; any situation will call up appropriate memories if it is once understood, i.e. if it is given meaning. The first is a more primitive type and is useful, even essential, for the innumerable, trivial adaptations of daily life. For instance, "Where did I leave my pen?" can be answered only by evoking the simple kind of isolated image memory. The laying down of my pen has no meaning beyond the me-ness attached to it. But "How did I begin this argument?" has objective meaning. This second type is a specialization of intellectual life and without it no intellectual achievement is possible. The first is childish, the second adult. With advancing age, "memory" gets poorer. This means that the primitive type is lapsing, the individual is approaching the state of a Korsakoff patient where new associations are not being formed, except in so far as they fit into existing patterns. As has been remarked before, some senile patients actually do develop the Korsakoff syndrome.

Bartlett has noted these two types in his paper on the Functions of Images, although calling them by different names. In the experiments there reported, he presented to his subjects series of picture-postcard photographs and signs arbitrarily associated with different simple words. Memories of this material were then demanded at different intervals after the original experience. He found that there were two types of subject which he called the visualizers and the vocalizers. In the former, the data were recalled preponderantly as images and the subject's confidence in the accuracy of his memory was proportionate to the vividness of the images. They were quite defective in reproducing the order of sequence in which the photographs had been shewn and were likely to transfer the signs from one word to another. The vocalizers, on the other hand, were apt to reproduce the data to themselves in the form of verbal descriptions, and tended to be doubtful of the validity of their memories: "They were prone to enter into long explanations and justifications of their attempted reproductions". They got more striking details, because at the outset they had picked out details that reminded them of something (that is,' they gave the details meaning when they first observed them). They could reproduce the order of sequence much better than could the visualizers. There were roughly as many mistakes in each of the two groups, but they were apt to be different kinds of error: while the visualizers invented new details, the vocalizers were apt to blend different data together. That is, the latter group manufactured meanings.

What Bartlett calls the vocalizer is a temperamental type that deals preponderantly with meanings. From study of my own memory capacity and incapacity I have concluded that I belong to this type. I have an unusually good memory for a few things and bad for most, and I have discovered that validity of memory with me is based on getting a meaning. From sad experience, I know that the meaning may be quite false, although that makes no difference at the time of my recall to the certainty I feel as to the reliability of the memory. If two data can be correlated in sense I am dangerously inclined to remember them as associated in space or time. In order to clarify this discussion, I may give an example of a false memory of my own which illustrates the mechanisms of both recall and judgment of validity.

The occasion was a luncheon party at which Mrs A. remarked that she had just finished reading Gibbon·aloud to her husband, and that they both regretted ending the monumental work. I remarked that this called to mind a literary allusion to someone who wept when he came to the end of Gibbon; but I could not recall the book in which I had read this nor its author. Another guest, Mrs B. (who has a remarkable and accurate memory for literary data), said that what I was thinking of occurred in Stevenson's essay *El Dorado*, but that she was not at all sure I had remembered the story correctly. Retrospectively she gave the items in her mind as follows: (1) an idea of ending a book, (2) a verbal image "no more worlds to conquer", (3) a visual image of something in quotation marks, and (4) a visual image of the part of the page where the passage occurred. I answered that I was sure that the story concerned Gibbon, but that I could not remember its having anything to do with Stevenson nor with *El Dorado*. We then looked up that essay and found the following:

"A young fellow recently finished the works of Thomas Carlyle, winding up, if we remember aright, with the ten note-books upon Frederick the Great. 'What', cried the young fellow, in consternation, 'is there no more Carlyle? Am I left to the daily papers?' A more celebrated instance is that of Alexander, who wept bitterly because he had no more worlds to subdue. And when Gibbon had finished the Decline and Fall, he had only a few moments of joy; and it was with a 'sober melancholy' that he parted from his labours."

One can see that I had here synthesized the three elements of finishing reading Carlyle, Alexander's tears, and Gibbon's completion of his writing. There is thus a meaning established; but it is not the meaning in Stevenson, nor in the present situation, but rather a combination of the two. Because the meaning is plausible, I am satisfied and feel the memory to be correct. Mrs B., on the other hand, keeps the elements separate and does so by retaining them as images.

Her feeling, or judgment, of validity was based on the clarity of the images, on the feeling of me-ness attaching to them and on their forming a unitary whole. This last is important. Without the congerie of images being given a local habitation and a name, they would have been merely images and not a "memory". If experience be called up as images, they cannot be rationalized, except as belonging to some localizable situation; they seem, like the thoughts of Claparède's Korsakoff patient, to be a fantasy of the moment. A meaning, however, can be rationalized in terms of the plausible. Hence, I can combine the same elements, or some of them, into a meaning and thus end the recall process.

Another kind of background process gives discrimination between fantasy or dream and real experience. The feeling of me-ness for a dream may be vivid, yet it is known to be a dream. There seem to be two types of discrimination employed. The first is the purely intellectual conscious judgment: the experience is impossible, therefore, it must have been a dream. For example, if I recall jumping over King's College Chapel, I have no hesitation in regarding this memory as a dream. The second is an automatic judgment that is based on associations of the recalled datum to its background. If the experience has a penumbra of associations with a wide range, it is held to be a real experience. We see examples of this both in the pathological liar and in the frequent case of a false memory, where a fantasy is given a setting from real life that would fit it, so that actual experiences may provide the penumbra. This latter kind of false memory can be frequently observed in the paranoid patient whose peculiar meanings justify the transference of a fantasy to some given situation. If, for instance, I fancy that a colleague has enmity towards me and says things derogatory of my character, I may imagine that he has spoken of me as a liar. Next, I recall seeing him conversing with another colleague last night, which may be a perfectly accurate memory. Then I place the word "liar" on his lips and it has now ample setting to justify it in my mind as a real memory. It naturally requires a dominating interest to manufacture the vital association.

If the experience recalled is inherently probable and the penumbra is limited, the judgment will depend on the apparent recency of the experience. This is because a recent, real experience ought to have a rich background of associations. If I recall meeting a friend yesterday in the market-place, I automatically call up a long series of associations: where I was going at the time, what I did thereafter, etc. If this extensive penumbra is present, I say that the recollection is of an actual event. If, however, it seems to have been an encounter within the last twenty-four hours and yet there is no memory for anything except it, no matter how inherently probable it may seem, I conclude it was a dream of last night. On the other hand, if images arise of my sitting in a railway carriage with a book on my lap and a man opposite with a beard and wearing a cap, and if this presentation carries no kind of time feeling with it, I am quite at a loss as to whether this really occurred some weeks ago when I was in a train or whether it was a dream. During these weeks, the natural lapse of unimportant associations would lead to an isolation in my mind of the central group of images, and realizing this, I hesitate either to affirm or deny that it was a rea experience.

One problem remains: why the certitude about the Battle of

Hastings occurring in 1066? The answer is somewhat tautological. It is a fixed association. It is like my certainty that "cat"
is the name for the animal known to science as *Felis domestica*.
It is not a case of voluntary recall but of eliciting a habit reaction
in which consciousness need not necessarily intermediate. We
accept all such fixed habit associations unquestioningly, for the
simple reason that no one questions them and that they do not
fail us in our daily adaptations. The acceptance of rigid habit
associations being generally useful, we extend this automatic
judgment of apodeictic certainty to all such associations. It is
for the same reason that the sight of a cat calls up the word "cat",
and that everyone knows what I mean by "cat", that I accept
the verbal association "Battle of Hastings 1066" as being equally
valid. It may, of course, be wrong; but the association is so immediate, it involves so little volition, that it *feels* right and I do
not bother to look it up. If, however, its accuracy were essential
to my argument, I would look it up before I put it in a book,
because I know my memory!

CHAPTER XIII

LAWS OF PATTERNS AS
DEDUCED FROM PSYCHOLOGY

I. When specific stimuli are applied to an organism synchronously or in immediate succession, each being of sufficient intensity to produce its appropriate reaction, there is a *tendency* for the reactions to become united together, *forming a pattern*. (Actually every known organism has, when first observed, a number of patterns already existing or potentially present. Were it not so the organism could not be recognized as such.)

(*a*) The first stage is a lowering of threshold for one or more of the stimuli. Past specific experience is here exerting an influence and this influence is called a liminal image. A chain of responses is thus formed.

(*b*) After sufficient repetition, the threshold falls to zero. Responses then occur to image functions.

(*c*) When a number of image functions are united in a pattern as an integrated whole, a new unit is formed, which may become a new image function acting as a unitary whole, just as a "perception" of subjective experience has a unitary quality.

II. *Functions of Images.*

(*a*) When an image function determines responses indirectly, which are not the specific reactions for it, it has become an image (objectively, the image has become a goal stimulus; subjectively, there is an awareness of a stimulus in the material absence thereof and without direct, specific response to it).

(*b*) Images function, therefore, to provide stimuli for programmes of activity rather than for single reactions. Programmes are an expression of personality, which, operating through consciousness, discriminates between images and perceptions. If this discrimination fails, the image acts as an hallucination.

In their operation images combine patterns. When this is effected, the combinations of patterns are adaptive to peculiarities of the situation. For this it is necessary to have a higher series of integrations (personality and consciousness) controlling reactions for which the image functions would be the appropriate stimuli. Without this control pathological reaction results.

From this we can reach the generalization that images or image functions are non-adaptive, unless controlled by higher integrations belonging to systems operating in response to stimuli of a different order from those to which the images or image functions belong. (Personality and consciousness deal with interests and meanings rather than perceptions: similarly, we might expect instincts to deal with projicient perceptions rather than with tactile stimuli.)

III. *Formation of new patterns independently of specific new experience.*

(*a*) Liminal images may allow utilization of substitutes.

(*b*) Images allow combinations of patterns. These, however, are unstable (deflection to actual goal). On the other hand, there must be instability to get modifiability, therefore, higher integrations are both more adaptive and more unstable, and more quickly established. The more primitive a reaction, the more repetitions are needed to establish it as a pattern. There is a reciprocal relationship between the necessity of repetitions and the capacity for the combining tendency.

(*c*) When images, or image functions, are well established, it is possible for patterns to be activated without external stimulus (interests) or, at least, in absence of stimuli specific for the unit patterns.

IV. *Activations of Patterns.*

(*a*) The appearance of a stimulus (disturbance external to central nervous system), duplicating an image or image function in a pattern, activates that pattern. The commonest stimulus is a metabolic or visceral state (appetite).

(*b*) Preliminary activation consists, we assume, in the reproduction of patterns in the form of liminal images. This lowers the threshold for environmental duplications of the imaginal material (attention), but raises it for stimuli of other patterns. Therefore, the activation of one pattern (or a series of allied patterns) involves the inhibition of other patterns not integrated therewith.

(*c*) When this occurs reaction takes place and thus, in so far as past experience is being represented, an image-function is operating. These are induced image-functions.

(*d*) This may also occur when a complicated pattern is strongly activated by one stimulus which sets the whole pattern going with such intensity that thresholds for its component elements are lowered to zero. These are spontaneous image-functions.

(*e*) When a stimulus activates one pattern dominantly, but subsidiary patterns are being activated by attendant stimuli, there is behaviour focussed on the object calling forth the dominant pattern and oriented by subsidiary patterns. This is perception. The nature of the reaction, as a whole, is determined by a dominant pattern, and is generic in quality.

(*f*) When reactions are focussed on an object but have their nature determined by attendant patterns, there is behaviour adaptive to the specific situation. This is meaning.

(*g*) No pattern can be activated without presentation of a stimulus duplicating an image conditioned therewith. (For example, images of attendant, orienting reactions cannot activate the central pattern, with which they were associated only in time, unless they have been conditioned with it. This comes about slowly by repetition of temporal association. When an attendant reaction mediates the central reactions, however, the association is not merely temporal but integral, and then conditioning may take place quickly, perhaps in one experience.)

(*h*) When a compound image function (of a perceptual order) is activated as part of a more complicated pattern, it appears as a unit and not in its component parts, because it is only as a unit that it has been integrated into a higher series of patterns. There is no connection between the elements in the subsidiary compound and the higher integration, but only between the latter and the subsidiary compound as a whole. For example, the sight of a cat calls up the word "cat" but never the letters a, c, or t. (This is a corollary to I (*c*).)[1]

(*i*) When a complicated pattern exists as a programme of activity, focussed on a given end, and having, as its *raison d'être*, reaction to that end, stimuli appropriate for the subsidiary patterns will not be effective in eliciting the total integrated pattern. The only effective stimulus for a "programme" pattern is the presentation of the goal towards which it tends. (This is a corollary to II (*b*).)

[1] This explains why consciousness does not normally control isolated visceral functions directly. It is only their general mass effects which are integrated with voluntary activities. This is a matter to be discussed in detail in a subsequent publication.

PART TWO

PHYSIOLOGICAL PATTERNS

CHAPTER XIV

THE BASIC FUNCTIONS OF
THE NERVOUS SYSTEM

IT might be said that the chief purpose of the present work is
to provide a vocabulary in which all the phenomena of living
matter can be discussed, enabling us to disregard the barriers
erected between the different branches of biological study. Expedience demands that such a huge field should be subdivided,
but an unfortunate result of the partition has been a separation in
point of view of workers in the different plots. Each has developed
his own vocabulary, and, consequently, has lost sight of the basic
principles common to all vital functions. The underlying unity
of the various sciences is expressed only in the adjective "biological". The comparative anatomist, or the physiologist, learns
little from, and teaches little to, the psychologist, because one
specialist has no means of expressing his findings in terms that
are significant for another specialist. However, if "patterns" are
common to the phenomena investigated in different laboratories,
the theory of patterns may be enlarged by any kind of biological
research. In order to establish the suitability of this terminology,
it would be necessary to demonstrate that the basic "laws" of
patterns as derived from psychology are just as much laws of
physiology or of embryology, for example. Within the confines
of one book it would be impossible to apply the theory in detail
to all branches of biology. I shall, therefore, confine myself chiefly
to physiology and, even there, to the physiology of the central
nervous system, making mention of its application in other fields
as such extension becomes apropos.[1]

It is usually stated that the simplest functions of nervous
tissue are analysable into irritability, conduction, and end-effect.
This triad, however, is found even in unicellular organisms, so it
is not peculiar to the nervous system. Jacques Loeb made many

---

[1] Except when otherwise stated, the data I am going to use are taken from
Sherrington's magnificent work, *The Integrative action of the Nervous System*.

experiments to shew the independence of alleged nervous functions
of any nervous system. For example, the jellyfish—medusa—
beats rhythmically. The margin of its "umbrella" contains
a ring of inter-connected ganglia; if this ring be cut off from the
rest of the body, the body as a whole ceases to contract, while the
ring containing the nervous tissue continues to do so. Loeb shewed,
however, that if the body containing no nervous elements were put
into water having a sufficient concentration of sodium ions it
would begin to beat again. But these beats were not co-ordinated
unless a bit of the ring were left attached to the body. Continuing
his investigations further he found that the remnant of nervous
tissue simply initiated a brisker contraction which then dominated
the whole bell. An analogous dominance of one portion of
contractile tissue over the rest of the mass was discovered in the
ascidian heart. This is nothing but a long tube in which waves of
contraction pass first one way and then another. Loeb shewed
that there were two centres, one at each extremity of the tube in
which contractions were initiated. Whichever one beat first
started a contraction wave that determined the pulsation of the
organ as a whole. (A centre in the sinus venosus in the frog's
heart operates similarly as a pace maker for the whole heart.)
Loeb found that two medusae joined together would beat as one
as a result of a similar dominance in rate of contraction of one
point which was transmitted to the grafted as well as to the original
body. An old experiment illustrating a co-ordinated movement in
the medusa is the application to one point of the sub-umbrella of
an irritating substance; the manubrium then moves to this point
as if to remove the irritant. Loeb gives a mechanical explanation
of this apparently purposeful behaviour, which is that the contractions set up from the irritated point are bound mathematically
to result in such a contraction as will bring the manubrium inevitably in the direction of the irritation—all this following from
the radial symmetry of the organism. This explanation breaks
down, however, for the case in which a cut is made parallel with the
margin of the bell and above the point irritated. This will obviously
interfere with the radiation of contractions from the irritated point.
If the protective reaction of the medusa be determined solely by
the principles of mechanics, the contractions in the mutilated
animal should direct the manubrium to a wrong point, but should
do so with the same certainty and invariability as is displayed in

the intact animal. Nevertheless, in this experiment the movements made by the manubrium are uncertain, as if it were searching for the irritant without sufficient information as to its whereabouts.

There can be no question but that Loeb has succeeded in demonstrating that apparently nervous functions can be mediated by contractile tissue without the aid of nervous tissue to conduct the impulses. It is notorious that much of the chemistry of the body is regulated by irritability, conduction and end-effect operating through the production and transport of chemical stimuli circulating in the body fluids. Such chemical stimuli have been called hormones, of which secretin furnishes an excellent example. This is a substance elaborated in the wall of the upper small intestine in the course of gastric digestion. It is then absorbed, passes into the blood stream and thus reaches the intestines lower down where it activates the secreting glands that function at a later stage of digestion.

These so-called basic nervous functions are, then, independent of any given type of structure, just as "flight" may be carried out by birds, bats, fish or aeroplanes. This would suggest that such functions are pattern activities. If so we should have to say that the structures mediate the functions but that they modify the functions as well. An analogy might be made with architecture: the architect's design is the ultimate determining agency for the form of a building which is achieved through the medium of different building materials; the nature of these materials will to some extent determine the design and affect the end result. The mere analysis of a structure on mechanical principles will not fully account for its functions any more than the study of the physics of a train will account for its behaviour. (I shall attempt to shew this presently for the central nervous system.) But it seems that there must be structures for the expression of patterns, and we observe that the more complicated and perfect a function becomes the more specialized is the structure through which it operates. This is a fundamental principle in evolution.

If irritability, conduction and end-effect can appear in the absence of nervous tissue what contribution do nerves make to such reactions? Loeb shewed that, when the same reaction can be carried out by an organism with or without its nervous system, the reaction in the former case is quicker and has a lower threshold. He demonstrated this very nicely in the ascidian *Ciona intestinalis*.

This lowly creature has a body roughly the shape of a fat sausage with two protuberances at one pole. The primitive gut of the creature runs from the extremity of one of these protuberances to that of the other, the two openings being called oral and aboral. Its nervous system consists of a ganglion in the crotch between the two protuberances. When the oral or aboral opening is irritated sufficiently the two protuberances contract and the animal assumes the shape of a ball. Loeb removed the ganglion, and then found that although the same reaction would take place it needed a much stronger stimulus to elicit it and the contractions were slow. Similarly, it has been found that when the iris of the vertebrate eye is severed from its nervous connections it will still contract but only in bright light and sluggishly. Again, some fresh water planarians have movements in detached aboral pieces when exposed to light but the movements are very slow.

From such experiments it becomes obvious that one of the functions of nervous tissue is to facilitate both the reception and the conduction of stimuli. What is not so obvious is a further effect that this must have on complicated movements. In order that these may take place co-ordinately, it is necessary that the stimuli for them should be transmitted to the moving parts with a speed much greater than that of any of the contractions. It follows, then, that co-ordination, depending on speed of conduction, will be dependent on the presence of nervous tissue, if the co-ordination be of movements that are at all rapid. Loeb cites some excellent illustrations of this. We have already in an earlier chapter referred to the capacity of the tail half of an earthworm to move in unison with the head half if the two halves be merely tied together with bits of thread. It is found, however, that a co-ordinated movement of the reunited worm occurs only when the front half moves slowly, once the latter speeds up the tail half will crawl at its own and slower rate. This shews us that the nervous system becomes an organ for expressing functions of the body as a whole. The principle is illustrated beautifully in the righting reaction of the starfish. If one of these creatures be placed on its back, two of its arms will twist over and seize the ground with its tube feet; having thus attached itself, the whole animal somersaults and thus regains contact for the whole ventral surface with the ground. If one arm be cut off and it be placed on its back, it will turn over: so mere turning over is a reaction independent of the nervous system. But if the nerve ring which connects the arms be cut, each arm will try to turn over by itself—co-ordination has disappeared. It is probably a safe generalization that no elaborate and rapid functions of an organism as a whole are conceivable without a nervous system, or at least without some similar structure having the properties of a nervous system.

From the experiments just cited one might conclude that of the three functions, irritability, conduction and end-effect, the nervous system in its specialization has chiefly elaborated that of conduction; that it has thus speeded up reactions but its functions are all ascribable to the algebraic sum of impulses that can be received and transmitted with great rapidity. If this were so the end-effect would always be dependent directly on the complex of stimuli at any moment and the functions of the nervous system would be passive. There are, however, a number of phenomena in quite simple spinal reflexes which indicate that the central nervous system does not operate as a simple machine, transmitting and transforming afferent into efferent impulses, but rather that special disturbances are set up within the central nervous system which issue as motor phenomena.

Before citing examples of these phenomena, it may be well to explain what a "spinal reflex" is. An animal such as a dog or cat has its spinal cord severed in the neck region, which means that there is a complete break in continuity between the head structures and the spinal part of the voluntary nervous system. After a period of "spinal shock", in which the animal lies flaccid and unresponsive, irritability in the limbs and trunk return. Various reflexes may then be elicited of which the chief ones studied have been the scratch reflex, flexion, crossed extension and extensor thrust. The scratch reflex consists of flexing a hind limb and then scratching at the flank with a series of flexions and extensions of the shortened limb; this reflex is elicited by irritation of a saddle-shaped area over the back and flanks, stimulation on one side always leading to scratching on the same side; the hind leg of the opposite side is frequently extended. The flexion reflex is a contraction of the muscles of all the joints of any one of the limbs drawing the limb as a whole up towards the body. The stimulus which produces this response is of a painful or harmful order (usually but not necessarily applied to the sole of the foot), and the reaction is therefore spoken of as nociceptive. The flexion reflex is studied as a rule in one of the hind limbs. When the flexion reflex is elicited in one hind leg, an extension in the opposite hind leg occurs with considerable regularity. This is known as the crossed extension reflex. The extensor thrust is an extremely rapid and powerful contraction of all the extensor muscles in a hind leg and it is elicited by firm pressure on the sole of that foot; ordinary electric or other nociceptive stimuli will not produce it.

The first phenomena to be considered in connection with these spinal reflexes are *latency* and *after-discharge*. When a stimulus is applied there is a latent period before reaction ensues and after the stimulus has ceased the response may continue for some time. Sherrington compares these peculiarities of the spinal reflex with inertia and momentum. Now, a simple reflex is supposed to be carried out by three organs, the receptor, the conductor, and effector. If, however, something in the central nervous system has to be set going and then, when going, proceeds by itself for a while, the central element has not merely the function of conduction but also of production. Something comes into being which produces the efferent impulses, so that these have no direct dependence on the stimulus whatever, originating rather in the "something" that appears in the central nervous system, which would be an impossibility if the function of the spinal cord were purely that of conduction.

The second phenomenon is the *summation of stimuli*: not infrequently a reflex may be elicited by a series of small stimuli any one of which, when acting alone, would produce no externally manifest effect. The explanation that Sherrington offers of this is that the first stimulus sets up an excitation facilitating the following one. This would presume that what is excited is the specific central mechanism, the same set of neurones that send out the final efferent impulses, but that these nervous elements are excited to a lower pitch of intensity than when discharge actually occurs. Were this group of cells operating in the same manner as they do when they emit efferent impulses (except for the moderate intensity), then we should expect this central disturbance to have a refractory period similar to that exhibited in the overt reflex. (See below for the description of refractory phase.) But Sherrington has shewn that the scratch reflex may be elicited by two subliminal stimuli, when the second falls in what ought to be the refractory period in the excitation set up by the first. The excitation of the scratch reflex is, moreover, not purely a threshold matter, for one single electric shock will never produce it, no matter how powerful it may be. On the other hand, "a single, brief, mechanical stimulation of the skin (rub, prick, or pull upon hair) usually succeeds in exciting a scratch reflex, though the reflex thus evolved is short; but there is nothing to shew that these stimuli, though brief, are really simple and not essentially multiple". The edge of a card laid evenly on the skin may not excite the reaction but an extremely light stroke along the same line will elicit it. The easiest way to generalize about effective stimuli for the scratch reflex is to say that they must resemble the effects of a parasite moving on the skin. This is quality. It is, perhaps, conceivable that a machine might be constructed to respond this way, but its complication would be almost incredible.

The third phenomenon is *rhythm of response*, such as appears, for instance, in the successive strokes of the foot in the scratch reflex. This is one of the best proofs of the function of the spinal part of the reflex arc being production rather than conduction of impulses, for the rhythm of the response is often markedly different from the rhythm of the stimulus. " . . . the rhythm of the end-effect indicates that in transmission along the reflex arc the impulses generated at the receptive end of the arc are not actually passed on from one cell element to another in the arc, but that new impulses with a different period are generated in the course of the reflex conduction."

Lastly, we may consider *refractory phase*. " . . . a state during which, apart from fatigue, the mechanism shews less than its full excitability." That is, there is a phase when, for that particular interval of time, only a very strong stimulus will produce an externally visible response or indeed it may be impossible to elicit any reaction whatever. Sherrington traces rhythmic responses to this factor: citing the case of the scratch reflex in which no stimulus, however strong, can produce a tetanus (that is, a prolonged continuous contraction). In other words, the excitability of the central mechanism is discontinuous. He also correlates the refractory period with the force of reflex movements. For instance, the extensor thrust is a powerful single contraction, lasting perhaps no longer than 170 thousandths of a second but with a refractory phase following it of a full second. The purpose of this is clearer than is the nature of the mechanism which could produce it.

Extensor thrust is a reflex essential to running with long strides. Following the thrust which raises and projects the body forward the animal sails through the air with flexed hind limbs and during the period of flexion, extension would of course be inappropriate. From the standpoint of patterns the phenomenon called refractory phase is highly important, for it introduces the element of time in the nature of the reflex response. It marks quality as well as quantity appearing on the efferent side.

From these examples we must conclude that, although the function of single nerve strands may be that of simple rapid conduction, when complicated organization of a central nervous system is encountered, processes are possible that represent an elaboration of something new, something that cannot be derived from a mere algebraic sum of in-coming stimuli. A basic function of the central nervous system is, then, this manufacture of specialized efferent impulses.

CHAPTER XV

IMAGINAL PROCESSES IN
NERVOUS FUNCTIONS

MANY attempts have been made to account for the functions of the central nervous system on the basis of mechanism, that is, structure operating solely on physical and chemical laws. These explanations are too technical to discuss here, but I may mention one difficulty characteristic of such interpretations. As Sherrington has abundantly proved, reflexes have a "double sign"; that is, when any given muscle or muscle group contracts, the muscles which would produce the opposite movement are not only inactive but their contraction is positively inhibited. This phenomenon is called "reciprocal innervation". Most theories make synapses (the junction points between anatomically separated nervous elements) responsible for inhibition. But in some invertebrates double sign occurs peripherally, that is to say, it occurs in continuous nerve trunks. The chorda tympani nerve in man may also transmit inhibitory impulses. Where are the synapses in nerve trunks? In general it is probably safe to state that no adequate mechanistic explanation of reflex phenomena has ever been achieved: no author can present such an hypothesis without another author appearing shortly after to prove that the explanation is *mechanistically* unsound. As the literature of neurology is replete with such criticisms, I shall not attempt to discuss the functions of the central nervous system mechanistically, but will endeavour rather to shew that the nervous system does things which no machine could do.

Mere intricacy of function is not impossible for a machine. The intricacy of an automatic telephone exchange, for instance, is staggering to the lay mind. But no machine has adaptability: it cannot change itself or its functions to meet new conditions, it does not improve its performance with practice, it cannot perform some particular function, depending originally on one part, after that part is destroyed. An internal combustion engine cannot learn by itself to run as well at a high altitude as at a low. If a motor-car turns in at a certain gate 999,999 times, it will have no more tendency to leave the road at that point the millionth time than it had the first. If one cylinder of a motor is put out of action, the speed and power of the engine is reduced in a mathematically predictable proportion; or the loss of a small part in a complicated mechanism may mean the total cessation of function, as in a watch that loses one wheel. Yet these are kinds of things which the central nervous system may do—or do without.

The non-machine qualities of the cerebrum are notorious and I need mention only one striking example. The early experimenters on the localization of function in the brain found that paralysis of one limb could be produced by excision of a small bit of the cortex in what is called the motor area. Unfortunately for the mechanists, however, it was soon found that, unless a really large amount of the brain were cut away, the function in the paralysed limb began to return after some weeks and might even be regained completely. The other wheels of the watch had, so to speak, taken on the job of the missing wheel. It is more interesting to examine spinal reflexes for examples of functions of a non-mechanical order, and I shall begin by considering phenomena that are adequately expressed in terms of patterns and imaginal processes. That is, I wish to direct attention to phenomena which seem to indicate the operation in the present of past experience which is not reproduced as a repetition of the stimuli coming from without the central nervous system. This, as I have argued, is the basic principle of conditioning or of Bahnung.

Liminal Images. If two independent reflexes utilize movements that have often occurred together, although belonging to quite different reflexes, there might be a tendency for these reflexes to be conditioned together. If so, the stimulation of one of these reflexes would tend to lower the threshold for the other. This is found to be the case in innumerable instances of which I shall give only one example. Stimulating either a front foot or hind foot produces flexion in the same limb. Having determined the threshold for this response in the hind limb, it is found that this reflex can be elicited with a subliminal stimulus if the crossed forefoot be stimulated at the same time. The probable basis for this conditioning is the coincident lifting of diagonally opposite limbs in walking—that is, a complicated reflex movement that has no other relationship to the simple flexion reflex. On the other hand, the flexion and scratch reflexes both include movements of flexion, yet they interfere with one another and do not reinforce. Flexion is here used towards different ends, it has different "meanings", that is, the succeeding reactions qualify it. Flexion that goes on to more flexion and flexion that goes on to clonic movements are quite different things and these different "backgrounds" make conditioning impossible.

Image Functions. When conditioning is complete, as we have seen, a reaction may be repeated in the complete absence of what was its original stimulus. An excellent example of this occurs in a co-ordination of eye muscle movements and the balancing apparatus in the inner ear which is known as the labyrinth. If a man rotates his head, stimuli are set up in the labyrinth which register the rotation. This may be consciously noted or may be deduced from the effects on distant muscles which regulate balance and movement. But, at the same time as the man turns his head, his eyes are moving too and hence things appear to move past him. Under such circumstances, we tend to follow the moving objects with our eyes, keeping one of them fixed in the centre of vision, and then, as the head has turned further round, to fixate at another point with a quick jerk of the eyeballs. The result is that the eyeballs make a series of short jerks in the plane of rotation, which is called nystagmus. Through countless experiences there has been a coincidence of labyrinthine stimuli with eye muscle movements so that the two have become integrated together. If, now, either the eye muscles or the labyrinth be stimulated alone the associated reaction in the other will tend to appear. For instance, if a man be placed in a whirling chair with his eyes closed and turned until he has lost control over his balancing reactions, it will be found that nystagmus is present in his eyes. Or, if hot water is applied to one ear and cold water to the other, although the subject's head is motionless, differential stimuli will be applied to the two labyrinths and the effects of rotation will be observed including not merely loss of balance (and dizziness) but also nystagmus. On the other hand, a susceptible person, while sitting in a train and moving at a constant velocity (without, therefore, receiving labyrinthine stimuli from the motion), who follows with his eyes the passing landscape and must accordingly employ nystagmoid movements, will become dizzy. That is, twitching of the eyeballs has produced the associated labyrinthine reaction. These illustrations are peculiarly forcible because the objective manifestations are parallelled by subjective imaginal experience. The subject, for instance, whose ears are being treated with hot and cold water reports that he feels as if he were whirling around at the same time that his eyeballs are moving, and the person who is dizzy often complains that things are whirling before his eyes and he feels as if they were so even if his eyes be closed. In other words, past experience is here being reproduced purely by association: reflex movements that I would ascribe to image function stimulation are produced, while at the same time the subject is consciously aware of these stimuli as images.

Sherrington gives some excellent examples of image functions in discussing what is known as local signature. A reflex is said to have local sign when its character is modified by shifting the point of stimulation. For instance, the scratch reflex exhibits local signature because the foot is always brought approximately to the point irritated. In such a case we are bound to assume that the afferent stimulus from the irritated point has a specific action in calling forth the particular reflex which directs the foot to that point rather than to another. In the performance of this reflex, however, specific afferent impulses have been generated in the muscles of the limb performing the movements. These two groups of afferent stimuli may then become so conditioned together that the correct response may be elicited in the absence of either one of them as the following examples from Sherrington will shew.

"The yellow clover fly will, after decapitation, stand cleaning its wings with its hind legs, and clean its 'three pairs of legs, rubbing them together in a determined manner, and raising its fore legs vainly in air as if searching for its head to brush up'...."

"In a reflex reaction exhibiting 'local sign' in the above sense, the afferent impulses involved are divisible into several groups according to their place of origin. There must be (1) a group originated at the seat of stimulus, (2) a group initiated in the motor and mobile organs reflexly set in action, and (3) in some cases a group arising at the distant spot to which the movement is directed. Regarding this last group an experiment illustrates its extinction without extinction of the 'local sign'. Thus, in Astacus, after section of the nerve-cords behind the mouth, when, therefore, the hind creature without mouth has lost all nervous connection with the front creature possessing the mouth, food given to the claws of the hind creature is still at once and accurately carried by them to the mouth, and this latter may refuse to take the morsel brought. In the grasshopper, after extirpation of the supra and suboesophageal ganglia (entire brain), the front leg is protracted, and in the normal way catches the antenna and the usual movements of cleaning the antenna go on, although the antenna has entirely lost its innervation owing to the destruction of the brain. Regarding the second mentioned group of afferent impulses, H. E. Hering has made the interesting observation that the 'cleansing' reflex of the spinal frog which brings the foot to a seat of irritation on the dorsal or perineal skin is accurately executed after severance of the afferent spinal roots of the limb itself. In the same way the bulbo-spinal frog brings the fore limb to the snout when the snout is stimulated after section of the afferent roots of the fore limb. The scratch-reflex I find executed without obvious impairment of direction or rhythm when all the afferent roots of the scratching hind limb have been cut through."

These illustrations of what I have been pleased to call image functions are concerned with the completion of relatively simple patterns, that is to say groups of reactions so closely integrated as to form fairly obvious units. There are, however, in the intact animal many responses which at times occur independently and at other times are co-ordinated with reflexes of distant parts. Simple reflexes which may thus fit in with each other are spoken of as allied. In the "spinal animal" these larger intergrations do not appear as such (for reasons to be given later) but apparently are still vaguely present in that there may be a spread of excitation from one to another of these simple allied reflexes. In our pattern terminology we would say that the reflex which is thus secondarily excited is aroused by an image function which belongs to the larger pattern of co-ordination.

Sherrington says:

"The more intense the spinal reflex—apart from strychnine and similar convulsant poisoning—the wider, as a general rule, the extent to which the motor discharge spreads around its focal area. Thus, as stimulation of the planta causing the flexion-reflex is increased, there is added, to the flexion of the homonymous hind limb extension of the crossed hind limb, then in the homonymous fore limb extension at elbow and retraction at shoulder, then at the crossed fore limb flexion at elbow, extension at wrist, and some protraction at shoulder; also turning of the head towards the homonymous side, and often opening of the mouth, also lateral deviation of the tail."

This is known as irradiation of which Sherrington says further: "Irradiation of a reflex attaches itself to the problem of the simultaneous combination of reflexes. It does so because it affords clear evidence that by irradiation a reflex assumes use of a number of final common paths that do not in the first instance belong to it, but belong in the first instance rather to reflexes arising in their own immediate segmental locality. From them a "reflex figure is formed". (A final common path is a path by which efferent impulses emerge to activate a specific group of muscles performing a simple reflex.) He then gives some excellent examples of the facilitation of one reflex by another, remarking, "...the reflexes whose effects are thus combined are always reflexes of what was termed above 'allied' relation". He adds, "Moreover, it seems to me significant that the irradiation extends rather *per saltum* than *gradatim*". This last point is of high theoretic importance, because it shews that the spread of excitation in the spinal cord does not proceed from neurone to neurone as a gradual infiltration, but rather that whole patterns are activated at once. Such patterns could, of course, be either anatomical or functional, a matter to which we shall be giving considerable attention. The important point is that allied reflexes may be activated without the presence of their specific exciting stimuli outside the central nervous system, and this is what I have called an image function activity.

Another interesting example of an image function is the stepping reflex which is best observed in the decerebrate dog. (This is an animal in which the higher brain centres have been cut off, leaving the spinal cord and brain stem in continuity. Such animals exhibit much more perfect postural reactions and can move so normally as not to appear unusual to an untrained observer.) If such an animal be suspended so that its paws are free from the ground, its legs hanging free, and one of the paws be then raised, the stretching of the extensor muscles of that leg from this passive movement will set up contractions in those extensors which lead in turn to an alternating contraction of the flexor muscles so that the limb moves up and down; this rhythmic movement is further transmitted to the other three legs, so that the animal "walks", although his feet are all in the air. Part of this total walking reflex may also be elicited in the spinal dog. If unipolar faradization be applied to one hind foot, the opposite hind leg will be extended and flexed with alternate rhythm. The rate of movement is constant, being quite independent of the strength of the stimulus. I should explain this by saying that the faradic current excites a flexion reaction in the same leg with which extension in the opposite leg is closely allied. The proprioceptive stimuli in the passively stretched flexor muscles in the crossed leg provide a stimulus for a highly co-ordinate movement natural only to the intact animal, i.e. walking.

It is a matter of great theoretic importance that the reflexes set up by irradiation may be incongruous—from the standpoint of the intact animal—with the original reflex. For instance, in the example quoted from Sherrington, when a flexion in one hind limb irradiates so that the crossed fore limb is protracted at the shoulder, flexed at the elbow and extended at the wrist, while the homonymous fore limb is extended at the elbow and retracted at the shoulder, the two front limbs are assuming positions appropriate for taking a step forward, while the two hind limbs are in a position appropriate to the maintenance of a fixed posture. If the animal were on its feet at such a time it would inevitably fall down. Before the theoretic significance of this inco-ordination is touched upon, it may be well to give some further examples of similar phenomena in spinal man.

During the war an opportunity was offered of studying the results of complete and incomplete severing of the spinal cord in healthy young men, whose general health—after the initial shock had subsided—was not greatly affected by the injury. The type of reflex disturbance then observed, which differs in some respects from the findings in laboratory experiments on animals, has been of great interest to neurologists. The data I shall quote are taken from the papers of Riddoch and Head.[1]

One characteristic of the "spinal" human being is that there are few simple "type" reflexes—few of the more or less discriminative responses associated with local signature. The tendency is, rather, for extensive irradiation to occur, so that massive movements take place. For instance, stimulation anywhere on the leg—and even on the abdominal skin—will produce a powerful, prolonged flexion of all the flexor muscles of the leg and extending to the abdominal muscles, that would flex the pelvis, and spreading even to the other side of the body. Such responses are called "mass reflexes".

[1] "The Automatic Bladder, Excessive Sweating and some other Reflex Conditions, in Gross Injuries of the Spinal Cord", by Henry Head and George Riddoch; "The Reflex Functions of the Completely Divided Spinal Cord in Man, Compared with those Associated with Less Severe Lesions", by George Riddoch. Both papers in *Brain*, vol. XL, parts 2 and 3.

One of the functions to which Head and Riddoch paid particular attention was the detrusor reflex of the bladder, i.e. the complicated co-ordination of contraction of the bladder wall with relaxation of the sphincters, which results in forcible evacuation of urine. It was found that, if the general health of the patient were good, the bladder would soon regain this function and fire off when the contained fluid reached a given volume. When they studied the variation in threshold (amount of fluid) for this reaction, some curious reciprocal relations with the mass reflexes became evident. These are of a kind that can be expressed readily in terms of patterns but are difficult to account for on any mechanistic basis.

The bladder was found to fire off prematurely (i.e. at a low threshold) under the following circumstances: When a mass reflex (operating through the isolated lower end of the spinal cord) is elicited; when a deep breath is taken; when the glans penis is pinched; when the rectum is distended with fluid by an enema; or even in one case, with a small area of anaesthesia around the anus, when that area was pricked by a pin. If one is prepared to admit the action of liminal images and image functions, a single explanation of all these cases is readily found. Under normal circumstances, the detrusor reflex occurs when the bladder is distended; distension of the bladder implies increase of pressure within the pelvis, and all these facilitating influences are associated directly or indirectly with increased pelvic pressure. In taking a deep breath, the diaphragm presses down on all the viscera necessarily including the pelvic ones. In flexor spasm the abdominal muscles contract and thus press on the viscera. The case of the full rectum needs no comment, but that pricking anaesthetic skin around the anus should produce a similar result is more surprising. Such pricking, however, elicits the superficial anal reflex, i.e. a contraction of the external sphincter. Normally, this contracts to retain the faeces in the rectum when, owing to their pressure, they tend to escape. Pinching the glans penis seems to work in an analogous way: it tends to excite the coitus reflex which includes contraction of the abdominal muscles.

It might be thought that there was an increase in hydrostatic pressure as a result of the reflex activities in the abdominal muscles and that the evacuation of fluid was, therefore, passive. This possibility was completely ruled out in Head and Riddoch's experiments. Moreover, the bladder would often fire off automatically when the end of the penis was swabbed off (for purposes of surgical cleanliness) before inserting a catheter and when no contractions of the abdominal muscles took place. Similarly, there could be no actual increase of pressure in the case where the anaesthetic skin around the anus was pricked. In these instances the increase of pressure was "suggested", so to speak, and could not possibly have been actually produced. That is to say, image functions of pressure were activated; and pelvic pressure, being the stimulus conditioned in normal life with micturition, elicited that reaction, although the tension within, and not without, the bladder is the normal specific stimulus for contraction of its walls.

Another curious point about these reactions is that both the coitus reflex and the defaecation reflex are alternative with urination and are, therefore, normally inhibited thereby. The association between the two lies in their possession in common of the element of pelvic pressure. Irradiation may thus produce incompatible reflexes because each contains a common element, just as, on the psychological level, prize fighting may lead one to think of a Beethoven sonata, both being performed in the Albert Hall. Head and Riddoch found that if, when the glans penis was irritated, erection occurred, the micturition was promptly inhibited. When once the reactions begin as real events, they inhibit one another because they use the same apparatus. I can think of the boxing match and of the Beethoven sonata, but I cannot experience them both at the same time.

Since the image function of pelvic pressure links the patterns for the mass reflexes with those for evacuation of the bladder, the irradiation can take place either way. Hence Head and Riddoch found that filling the bladder or the rectum with fluid, or the act of spontaneous micturition, might evoke flexor spasms. Sometimes only the great toe would move upward. This last is peculiarly interesting. It is the simplest and most primitive element in the total flexion reflex, the purpose of which is to remove the foot from a harmful stimulus. But, when this slight movement takes place, there is, of course, no participation of the abdominal muscles. A long train of image functions must then be in operation. Moving the foot is associated with raising the leg, the latter with flexing the pelvis through contractions of the abdominal muscles; this is conditioned with heightened pressure in the pelvis and the last with the detrusor reflex. There are then four steps unrepresented in any overt action.

A most interesting case was one of partial lesion of the cord shewing total loss of control of micturition, excessive mass reflexes, and only a partial loss of sensibility. One side of the body was analgesic, i.e. insensitive to pain stimuli, which are the normal excitants for the flexion reflex. Pin pricking on either side would produce extensive flexion responses; but only when this stimulation was applied to the analgesic side did it facilitate urination. The significance of this is that the image functions set up by any reflex produce pathological results only when the control of higher integrations is lacking. The purpose of an image function is to combine patterns. This combination contributes to the behaviour of the organism as a whole and is irrelevant to the behaviour of localized organs. When, therefore, an image function activates another pattern of localized function and not a large co-ordinating pattern the result is inco-ordination; it is non-adaptive. This is law II (b) of our psychological patterns.

So far I have tried to demonstrate that the central nervous system operates on the principle of patterns, involving reproductions of past experience which would be impossible in a machine. This view is not really new for it is implicit in Head's doctrine of "vigilance".[1] This he defines as a kind of physiological efficiency: "The extent to which the activities of a particular portion of the central nervous system exhibit at any moment signs of integration and purposive adaptation indicate its vigilance". Variations in vigilance he believes to be the product of physical factors: "Vigilance is diminished, not only by structural changes in the central nervous system, but also by toxic influences such as chloroform, sepsis, or anything which tends to lower physiological capacity". But the functions which are so altered have just those properties which I have been describing as pattern activities. "In all specific modes of behaviour, conscious and automatic processes are inextricably mingled. Normal sensation demands not only recognition of qualitative and spacial differences, but also accurate registration on a physiological level of the result produced by previous afferent impressions." (It should be men-

[1] "The Conception of Mental and Nervous Energy: Vigilance, a Physiological State of the Nervous System", *Brit. Jour. Psychol.* vol. XIV, p. 126.

tioned that Head's use of the term "conscious" is roughly equivalent to the layman's word "mental".) "Purposive adaptation is
more or less evident in all responses, somatic or psychical, which
occur in a high state of neurone vigilance.

"Three factors are responsible for this character in the response.
Firstly, certain qualities in the stimulating object are ignored, whilst
others give rise to a reaction; these reactions in turn struggle among
themselves for mastery and their final integration gives significance to
one aspect of the stimulus rather than to another. Secondly, the form
assumed by the response at any moment depends on dispositions due
to past activities, and the future is implicit in the present. Thus the
behaviour of the central nervous system, in whole or in part, becomes
an orderly march of events and is not a series of isolated episodes.
Thirdly, afferent impulses endow the response with spacial relations:
the resultant action is co-ordinated to a definite end in space and in
time."

We should note that Head here describes physiological processes
in unequivocally psychological terms such as purpose, discrimination, "future implicit in present". This last is particularly interesting, in that it implies imagery of some sort. Mechanistic physiology, on the other hand, describes processes in terms of physics
and chemistry, of which an excellent example in A. V. Hill's
account of the processes in muscular contraction. Head does not
confuse psychology and physiology unwittingly: he says the two
are really one. "Mind is the resultant of a number of forces,
which culminate in both conscious and unconscious activities.
Once generated, these interact, producing a continuum in space
and time. But analysis of the behaviour they produce shews that,
from the highest to the lowest, they exhibit certain characters in
common, which depend on qualitative selection, duration and
projection."

CHAPTER XVI

MECHANISTIC EXPLANATIONS

HEAD's formulations could be put into terms of patterns operating with the co-operation of images and image functions. We should then say that, when the central nervous system exhibited vigilance, patterns were already activated to a liminal image level so that given functions were facilitated. On the other hand, when he speaks about the factors that cause a variation of vigilance, he emphasizes an indisputable fact that physical conditions affect the efficiency of operation of these patterns. Chloroform, for instance, will knock out the higher integrations progressively, and these will return again in order as the anaesthetic is eliminated from the body. Not only poisons have such effects. Gross injuries, inflammations or degenerations will modify or abolish functions. In fact diagnosis in "organic" neurology is based on theories of correlation of function with structure, and is often remarkably accurate. Such successes have fostered the hope—and even fortified the faith—that all functions can be translated adequately into terms of physical and chemical processes operating with and through material structures. We must now examine this type of interpretation in order to determine what the facts are to which our theories must be adapted.

In the main, the large conduction tracts in the central nervous system have been accurately mapped out and their functions determined with reasonable certainty. The necessity for these tracts, as specific channels of communication between different points in the central nervous system, seems to be almost as complete as in that for the maintenance of a wire connecting two distant telephone exchanges. In the grey matter of the cord, brain-stem and brain—which corresponds more to the telephone exchange itself, in which connections and cross connections are made—the dependence of function on specific regions of structure is much less certain. It is true that a number of "centres" have been identified and localized; these, however, are apt to have shifting boundaries and their functions can often be assumed vicariously by other parts. But, even if we assume that a given function is localized in some centre, how are we to envisage, in mechanical terms, the processes that go on there? How does the energy of a stimulus become transformed into specific efferent impulses producing various reflexes? If the nerve fibres were like the wires and terminals in a telephone exchange, that could be physically moved so as to make various connections, the problem would be theoretically simple. Unfortunately, no mechanist has even had the temerity to suggest that the terminations of the nerve fibres might actually move so as to establish various series of connections. The attempts that have been made have been rather in the direction of assumptions of changes in resistance in different strands of a nervous network, which might result in a re-arrangement of the impulses entering that network. Physiologists have been searching, therefore, for some structure in the course of nerve fibres or fibrils which might offer varying resistance to the nerve impulses passing along them. For many years the faith of the physiologist was in the existence of synapses, which might have the required physical attributes; more recently, theoretical attention has been turned to regions of decrement.

The doctrine of synapses originates in the study of neurones, i.e. the separate cell elements making up the purely nervous tissue in the nervous system. There are two chief sources of the evidence for the existence of separate nerve elements rather than of a syncytium in the composition of the brain spinal cord. (A syncytium is a confluence of cells which are so merged over one into the others that no boundaries can be detected between them anatomically.) The first source is embryology: in the course of development it is seen that the nerve cells are entirely separate, many of them develop *in situ* and others migrate to their proper localities, and then send out long processes which extend to other parts of the central nervous system or emerge as the fibres composing the peripheral nerves. The evidence for the continued separation of these elements is that if a nerve process be cut it will degenerate to the end of the fibre but will not affect the life of the other cell elements with which it has been in functional contact. Assuming, then, that the nervous system is made up of anatomically separated units, these cell elements have been divided into three main groups: afferent cells, whose processes carry sensory impulses into the central nervous system; efferent cells, which convey impulses away from the central nervous system to glands or muscles; and connector neurones, which somehow collect, re-arrange and transfer to the efferent neurones the impulses coming in on the sensory side. The hypothetically most simple reflex contains an afferent, a connector and an efferent element, but the behaviour of reflexes is such as to make it impossible that a single connector neurone could produce the observed results alone. It is, therefore, assumed that, with even the simplest reflex, a considerable number of connector neurones is involved. These connectors are sometimes spoken of as internuncial neurones or as making up internuncial paths.

At the junctions between the functionally connected termini of the cell processes belonging to different neurones are the synapses. Careful histological examinations have shewn nerve fibrils ending in a variety of branched arborizations or basket-shaped swellings. These so-called synaptic endings lie in juxtaposition to other cells or analogous terminal branchings of the processes of the latter. What the nature of the actual connection may be remains a matter of pure conjecture. Some have suggested that there are unstainable membranes interposed between the synaptic endings, others that there is really a continuity of fibres which, again, cannot be stained by any known technique, while still others think that there is a continuity of fibres which merely suffer a constriction at the synaptic junctions. So far as actual observations go, we are forced to assume that functionally a connection does exist for the simple reason that impulses are, quite obviously, transferred from one part of the nervous system to another. On the other hand, the time relations of excitation and discharge in the simplest reflex shew a very much longer interval than would be required for the transmission of a nervous impulse travelling the distance it has to go, if the impulse could travel through the central nervous system with the speed it is known to have in a nerve trunk. There is, therefore, some kind of a block within the central system and it has often been ascribed to synaptic resistance. Until there can be some demonstration of the mechanical nature of the disturbance in the connector neurones which manufactures the efferent discharge, the rôle played by the synapses must remain purely hypothetical. According to such hypotheses the synapses operate like one-way valves, or as selective filters inhibiting, reducing, or admitting impulses, so as to direct them to the final common path. Evidence being completely lacking as to the physical nature of the synaptic connection, these hypotheses are really tautological: instead of saying "mechanisms in the internuncial neurones", the neurologist says "selective action of the synapses". It has recently been pointed out that the all-or-none law, so well established for the arousal and propagation of an impulse in the peripheral nerve fibre, is inconsistent with the reduction of intensity that is presumed to take place in passing through a synapse: if this law held within the central nervous system, an impulse might be reduced in passing through a synapse but would promptly jump to its full potential on getting past the block. We should, therefore, have to assume that synapses could only block or admit impulses. If they blocked the transmission of impulses through certain portions of a nervous network, a specific arrangement of impulses emerging from the network could be achieved. This would, however, be an absolutely rigid system giving unvarying responses: for instance, it is difficult to see how inhibition could be lifted with such an arrangement. As a matter of fact, synapses are now falling into disrepute with physiologists, when considered as sole selective agencies in the re-arrangement of nervous impulses.

Before going on to consider the decremental region theories, we must first glance at the subject of the nerve impulse, without a knowledge of which speculation as to the functions of the nervous system are idle. This has been the object of a large amount of research in the last twenty years, which, with its exquisite technique, has presented a body of facts so definite as to make them the inevitable basis of all mechanistic speculations. The nerve fibre within the central nervous system can, of course, not be isolated for study, but the peripheral nerve fibre may be and, since the introduction of such fine physical apparatus as the string galvanometer, its electrical properties have been subjected to the closest scrutiny.

Conduction is present in plants as well as in animal tissues. Lillie[1] has brought forward arguments to shew that it is probably of the same fundamental nature in all living tissues. It is, however, best studied in the peripheral nerve fibre which has been specialized for this function. A large body of observations seems to shew that a stimulus—whether mechanical, electrical, thermal or what not—

[1] *Physiological Reviews*, 1922, vol. II, p. 1.

when applied to the nerve fibre, produces there some local disturbance. This local disturbance in turn generates an impulse that travels along the fibre, being detectable in its course as a wave of negative electrical potential, which can influence an electrode placed on the surface of the fibre. It has also been demonstrated that carbon dioxide is given off by the nerve during the process of conducting impulses. A point of fundamental importance we owe to the experiments of Adrian. He found that, in the isolated fibre, the strength of the impulse, once it was set up, remained constant and could not be increased by augmenting the strength of the stimulus. This is known as the all-or-none law of the nerve impulse. It has further been shewn that, when a given spot has just transmitted the impulse, it is for a short period of time incapable of producing or transmitting another impulse: this is known as the refractory period. Following the refractory period again, there is another short stage of hyper-excitability—at least this phase is present when the fibre is immersed in a weakly acid medium.

Lillie, who has given the most complete account of conduction in electrical terms, compares the phenomena to those observable in an iron wire covered with a coating of oxide and placed in a bath of nitric acid. If the coating of oxide is scratched so that the nitric acid gains a contact with the wire a miniature electric battery is formed, the bare portion being the anode and the neighbouring oxide film the kathode. The electric current thus engendered causes a reduction at the cathode and a re-oxidation at the anode. The part where reduction has taken place is again oxidized at the same moment that a still further point is being reduced. There is thus produced an oxidation and reduction in adjacent points in the wire that travel like a wave along the course of the wire, and this pair of chemical changes is dependent on the electrical circuit set up where one portion of the iron is originally exposed to the nitric acid. In such a case, the speed of the impulse depends on the speed of the disintegration of the oxide coating, while the capacity for transmitting repeated waves depends on the speed with which re-oxidation can take place. Lillie argues that a semipermeable membrane between fluids of different ionic concentration will give the same phenomena, i.e. a wave of polarization. He shews, further, that such a structure would finally respond to a summation of sub-minimal stimuli and, in fact, would produce all the phenomena that have been observed in isolated nerve fibres. This theory, then, is now pretty generally accepted by physiologists: the nerve impulse is considered to be a progressive wave of polarization brought into being by the passage of ions through a semi-permeable membrane that insulates two fluids of different ionic concentration.

The electrical theory of conduction of impulses seems to receive more confirmation every day, so we are probably safe in assuming its truth. Physiologists nowadays assume further that there is no essential difference in kind between the impulses in the peripheral and in the central nerve fibres. On this basis, they try to fabricate hypotheses of central nervous system function that will eliminate the notion of qualitatively different nerve impulses within and without the central nervous system. To assume qualitatively different impulses, is, of course, almost tantamount to admitting functions that cannot be put into terms of physics and chemistry: the ascription of the quality becomes mere tautology—as physiologists well know. A theory, however, which accounts for phenomena in terms of the interaction of definite physical or chemical units, that are of a measurable order, is not tautological. An excellent example of such an hypothesis is that resting on the well-established phenomena of conduction with decrement.

This theory was first suggested by Adrian and Lucas and has been more recently elaborated by Forbes[1] with great ingenuity. If a portion of a nerve fibre be exposed to the right dosage of chloroform or some other toxic agent, instead of transmitting impulses undiminished (according to the all-or-none law), they will suffer a gradual extinction; stronger stimuli, however, may succeed in forcing an impulse through the decremental region, when it will at once regain its standard strength on reaching the normal tissue. A most important phenomenon appears in studying the effects of a summation of stimuli on a decremental region. If the successive stimuli fall on the refractory periods of previous impulses, they are extinguished and nothing gets through. If, however, they fall on the periods of hyper-excitability ensuing on the refractory phase, their potency is augmented, and such impulses will penetrate through the poorly conducting zone. It was the discovery of this that provided Keith Lucas with an explanation

[1] *Physiological Reviews*, 1922, vol. II, p. 361.

of the so-called Wedensky effect, which is that, when a nerve muscle preparation has been stimulated to the point of fatigue so that no more contractions of the muscle occur, if the rate of stimulation be reduced, contraction may re-appear in the muscle. Lucas argued that a region of decrement existed at the neuro-muscular junction; at the original rate of stimulation, the impulses were falling on the successive refractory periods in this region; when the rate was reduced, the impulses fell after the refractory periods had ended.

On the basis of this explanation, a theory of reciprocal inner-vation was suggested by Adrian and Lucas. The phenomenon of reciprocal innervation is that when extensor muscles are in con-traction the opposing flexors are not merely inactive but are posi-tively inhibited of response. The proposed mechanism is illus-trated in Fig. 1. *A* is a nerve fibre running to a muscle which is

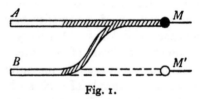

Fig. 1.

going to be inhibited. *B* is a fibre running to a muscle which will contract. A side branch runs from *B* to *A*, so that after their point of junction the nerve fibre to *M* would carry the sum of the im-pulses from both *A* and *B*. According to the theory, this last portion of the fibre (or the synapse at which the coalescence takes place) conducts with a decrement, so that the impulses from one source fall in the refractory period of the impulses from the other, and, in consequence, no impulses from either source can get through.

Forbes has elaborated this explanation to account for the major, classical phenomena of reflexes in the spinal animal: he invents numerous cross connections and relay paths, which would produce the necessary interferences that are actually observed. The reader is referred to Forbes' paper for a detailed description of the theory, that can only be explained here in the general principle I have just given. The scheme is, of course, complicated, but histological observation reveals a capacity on the part of the nerve fibres within the spinal cord for cross connections of a bewildering complexity: so complexity is no argument against his hypothetical mechanism. There are naturally various minor criticisms that can be levelled at Forbes' reconstruction, but these could probably be got round by assuming further accessory paths to account for neglected phenomena. I shall, therefore, raise only certain general objections.

Referring to Fig. 1, we can see that if impulses started together from A and B (or, indeed, if they started from either one of them first), at least one impulse would get through to M before the crowding and blocking took place; there should, therefore, be an initial twitch in the muscle before it is inhibited. This is in fact what occurs in the Wedensky phenomena. The first application of the stimulus to the fatigued nerve-muscle preparation produces a single twitch after which the muscle becomes unresponsive. But such an initial twitch is never observed in spinal reflexes when they are inhibited; in fact, Sherrington reports that inhibition may be so prompt as actually to precede the associated reaction of excitation. My imagination fails to encompass a system of paths which produces inhibition as the result of regions of decrement inserted in the network, when the inhibition anticipates the positive discharge.

In order to account for the dominance of flexion over extension in the spinal animal, Forbes assumes that more neurones lead up to the extensor premotor neurones (the ones that pass impulses on to the final motor neurone), increasing the likelihood of raising the frequency of impulses at this synaptic junction above the critical point. When one considers the postural influences affecting these reflexes, a difficulty arises that seems to me insuperable. Forbes offers an explanation only for what is called postural reversal. The experimental fact is that if a limb be already extended, stimulation may lead to flexion, while if the limb be already flexed, extension may take place. He assumes that shortening (either active or passive) in extensor muscles sets up proprioceptive impulses, and that these are sufficiently slow in rate to be below the critical frequency in the extensor premotor synapse. (As a matter of fact, proprioceptive stimuli, that elicit reflex response, seem to arise much more from tension, active or passive, in the muscle and its tendons than from shortening. This, of course, would throw Forbes' explanation of postural reversal out of court.) The return of proprioceptive stimuli from the contracted muscle tend to perpetuate the extension, which is the "shortening reaction" of postural tone that Sherrington has described, and is a prominent feature of decerebrate animals. According to Forbes, the extensor premotor neurone is now receiving about all the impulses it can transmit without mutual interference. If a further stimulus is thrown in, the critical point is past, so that what has been excitation in the extensor premotor neurone becomes inhibition. On the other hand, if the limb be already flexed, there are no such proprioceptive impulses crowding in on the extensor premotor neurone, so that an appropriate stimulus reaching it causes the necessary excitation for extensor response.

Now, although there are some postural effects observable in the spinal preparation, the bulk of them appear in the decerebrate or intact animal. The chief influence determining postural effects must, therefore, come from, or be associated with, the neural mechanisms of the higher centres. How can these be attached to Forbes' scheme? If the higher centres throw impulses into the lower neurone system as he represents it, the effect will always be to increase the frequency of impulses above the critical point at those junctions where most neurones already converge, i.e. at the extensor premotor neurones. The effect of higher influence would then be inevitably towards inhibition of extension. As a matter of fact, just the reverse is true. In the decerebrate preparation, extension tends to dominate over flexion and such an irrelevant stimulus as a loud sound seems to increase the general excitability of the central nervous system and may throw the animal into extensor rigidity. We must, therefore, conclude that a scheme like Forbes' might explain many of the reactions of the spinal animal, but that a totally different scheme becomes necessary when the animal is decerebrate or intact. Yet, the section of the central nervous system axis which isolates the bulk of the spinal cord does nothing anatomically to the lower centres.

This is but an example of objections that may be made on more general grounds. Forbes' scheme represents a rigid system depending for its effects on a fixed series of rates of impulses in the various neurones. Such a system might work well enough in total isolation from outside influence, but would be dislocated from its normal function completely if more impulses were thrown into it than those arising from its own afferent nerves. This would mean that the system could not be taken over to become part of a larger system. Yet all the evidence goes to shew that spinal reflexes are merely modified when integrated in the service of the body as a whole. Interference from without in Forbes' scheme would mean reversal of reactions, not modification.

Forbes disclaims the probability and only alleges possibility for any scheme of the kind he had devised. But two notorious phenomena make any mechanical scheme impossible: these are vicarious function and perfecting with practice. In a machine, a weak link does not improve with use but wears out faster as the strain is prolonged. Yet, in the recovery from spinal shock (which we shall be considering a little later), the crossed extension reflex takes some time to recover and, while still weak and fitful, is much improved by practice. In explanation of this Forbes adopts Pike's theory that this reflex normally involves paths to the brain and back again, and modifies this view " ...to the extent of assuming in the intact nervous system a functioning connection between the local afferent and motor neurones, but one with a decrement so great that the summation effect of impulses from the brain is required to overcome it, and further assuming, in the gradual change known as recovery from shock, a decrease in the degree of decrement enabling the same spinal connection to conduct even without this reinforcement." Now, it has been abundantly proved that the phenomena of spinal shock are not dependent on nutritional influences, but are concerned with some kind of a re-arrangement of purely nervous functions. If, as Forbes assumes, decrements are subject to variations apart from nutritional and toxic changes, what becomes of their specificity—a specificity which is fundamental to mechanistic theories of the kind he favours?

CHAPTER XVII

ANATOMICAL DESIGNS

BEFORE we can go further in discussion of patterns at the physiological level, it will be necessary to arrive at some kind of an understanding as to the reciprocal relationship of structure and function within the central nervous system. I shall assume that purely mechanistic hypotheses are untenable; but, on the other hand, it is impossible to neglect the fact that functions are grossly modified when certain changes take place in the structures within the central nervous system. It is, therefore, necessary to devise some formulae which can take into account both the structural and functional factors at the same time. We must first see what is the nature of the previously irreconcilable facts that have to be harmonized.

Without question, the co-ordination of movements in different parts of the body depends on the integrity of tracts which unite the innervations of separate regions of the body. These paths of communication compose the white matter of the central nervous system. On the other hand, in the generation of co-ordinations, impulses are received by certain sensory channels, are then somehow re-arranged and emitted by motor nerves to the glands and muscles performing the co-ordinated function. This re-arrangement seems to occur in various more or less well defined areas of the grey matter that are spoken of as centres for the functions in question. The regions of neural interconnection have a wide and varying distribution and, moreover, in varying amounts of grey matter, sufficient connection can be established between afferent impulses and efferent discharges specific for given reflex movements. Partial destructions of a "centre" will not permanently destroy its function. From these facts it would, therefore, appear that our scheme must allow for complete dependence on structure, so far as intercommunication of distant parts is concerned, but that the dependence of the actual manufacture of specific correlated efferent discharges on structure is much looser.

Excitation, particularly over-excitation, of one reaction in the spinal animal may lead to the activation of others which have never been co-ordinated with it in normal life. If specific reactions depend on the excitation of specific neurones, then we are probably justified in saying that the neurones belonging to unit reactions never co-ordinated together do not form parts of any large self-contained constellation of neurones. For example, micturition and coitus never occur together and, therefore, are never co-ordinated: the groups of neurones, whose excitations presumably give rise to these reactions, cannot belong to any larger system of neurones whose function it is to produce coitus and micturition combined. The only anatomic connection that could exist between these two would be that each contained an element in common, i.e. that both the coitus neurones and the micturition neurones had the same sub-group of nervous elements which registered or represented the stimuli arising from pelvic pressure. A further difficulty to be reckoned with is that the interrelations of such inco-ordinated reflexes vary quite obviously from time to time.

The absence of continuity of the spinal cord with the higher centres seems to facilitate a random and, apparently lawless, series of connections between lower centres. On a mechanical basis, we should have to assume that the energy, which in the intact nervous system went to the higher centres, is dammed up in the lower ones, and so overflows to neighbouring lower centres. If a nerve impulse depends on a difference of potential between insulated electrolytes, a break in the insulation (cutting the fibre) could hardly lead to a larger difference of potential being reflected back from the break, particularly, if it had to return along a path including synapses, where impulses are supposed to travel only in one direction!

Only a system working on the basis of quite unknown physical principles could give these results. We must look, therefore, for some formulation which admits and combines both mechanistic and immaterial factors, each having its own rôle to play. Naturally, any hypothesis that can be fabricated at present must necessarily be highly speculative, particularly since there have been so far practically no observations made directly on the intimate events within the central nervous system itself. It seems extremely improbable that experimental ingenuity could ever succeed in dealing with the physics and chemistry of the microscopic elements within the brain and spinal cord without creating such disturbances as would hopelessly pervert the function of these structures. If this be so, all hypotheses as to what goes on within the central nervous system must remain a matter of inference from what can be observed to go into it and come out. The value of these hypotheses can only be judged by the extent in which they may succeed in correlating and rationalizing a larger and larger body of phenomena.

Let us begin with a further consideration of the basic properties of nervous tissue. Stimulation, conduction and end-effect compose the essence of nervous function. These may be present without a nervous system and, as Loeb has shewn, the advent of specialized nervous tissue brings about lowered threshold and greater speed of conduction and, therefore, greater speed in the ensuing reactions. What he did not see (or at least did not emphasize) was that these factors make possible a third development, namely new co-ordinations. The function of every complicated mechanism depends on the simultaneity or succession of movements in its parts. The speed of the slowest of them will set a limit to the complication of performance of which the mechanism is capable. For instance, bells take a long time to swing and return to their normal position, and they are, therefore, only capable of primitive musical effects. No mechanical device for enabling a man to pull many bells at once, or to pull more quickly, would make them capable of playing piano music, so long as the bells had to swing. But, if the bells were struck with small rapidly moving hammers and their vibrations damped, some pretence at reproduction of piano music might be achieved. A better example is, perhaps, the engine of a motor car. In this explosive gas is ignited by heat. The method of producing this heat rapidly and at the precise moment when the gas is compressed is the *sine quâ non* of the modern internal combustion engine. We might imagine the heat to be produced by friction; a cumbrous apparatus would then produce the heat slowly and much energy would be absorbed by the ignition apparatus. A further advance would be the introduction of something like a match; the apparatus would still be cumbrous and slow, but it might conceivably work in a low speed engine. Finally, an electric spark is used as the source for the heat, and is produced by a special apparatus, the magneto; the energy involved is now negligible and accurate timing of explosions makes possible the integration of many cylinders. An important point to be noted in this analogy is that with the development of greater speed there is also an economy of energy expended in the production of a specialized stimulus.

The same kind of effect is observable in the central nervous system. Rapidity in the contraction of muscles is quite futile without rapid conduction in the nerves which makes possible highly co-ordinated, concerted and segmental movements in the four limbs, the head and eye muscles, and so on. The most fundamental element in the co-ordination is the speed of conduction.

What is the nature of the specialization which brings this about? According to the modern electrical theory of conduction, there are two processes involved in the production and propagation of impulses: there is a permeation of an insulating wall placed between electrolytes of different concentration and a restoration of the equilibrium by the building up of the barrier once more. The effect of the stimulus—no matter what its physical nature may be —must be to reduce the effective resistance in the insulating membrane; and stimuli will differ in their efficiency according to the degrees in which they achieve this single result. Naturally, there are two ways in which penetration may take place. The continuity of the membrane may be broken by mechanical means, or the difference of electrical potential on the two sides of the insulation may be altered. The latter would probably involve less expenditure of energy, which accounts for the facility with which an electrical stimulus induces a response in a nerve fibre and the relative indefatigability of the nerve fibre stimulated electrically— the barrier membrane is not grossly injured.

If the repair phase—the stage during which the barrier is being replaced—were as rapid as the dissolution of the membrane, no change in the insulating capacity of the membrane would appear. The stimulus must, therefore, effect a lowered resistance more quickly than the resistance can be re-constituted. The properties of the membrance can, therefore, be inferred from the intensity and duration of an effective stimulus. On the other hand, were the repair phase very slow, it would be a long time before the system was again produced in which the two electrolytes of different concentration were once more insulated one from the other. Until the system is again reconstituted, the nerve fibre is incapable of producing and propagating an impulse; this is probably the refractory phase and its duration would be a measure of the speed of the repair process. An efficient nerve fibre will have a membrane whose electrical resistance is quickly reducible and almost as quickly re-established; such a fibre can propel many impulses per second. (The measured numbers are three hundred to one thousand per second in peripheral nerves.) It would seem that the nature of this membrane is the all important factor in the specialization of nervous tissue.

Primitive tissues are capable of all functions. Specialization involves a reduction of all but one function and performance of it with a greater efficiency, i.e. greater speed and at the expense of less energy. If the functions of the membrane be to protect from mechanical injury, it must be thick, tough, and relatively inert. Its constant repair would mean a gross physical accretion of matter. But a membrane which separates fluids of nearly the same ionic concentration can vary its functions with a slight change of electro-chemical constitution, involving a very slight expenditure of energy. Once such a specialized membrane is developed, a minute increase of ionic concentration at one point will start a wave by producing penetration in a membrane that is designed to insulate against only slight differences of potential. This is a specialized stimulus. A non-specialized stimulus will be effective only in so far as it contains, or produces, this specific element. Consequently, there may be a vast disproportion between the energy display of an artificial stimulus and the energy exhibited in transmitting an impulse along a nerve fibre, or in passing it from one fibre to the next.

It is, therefore, probable that within the central nervous system impulses are propagated more efficiently than in peripheral nerves. The latter live in a more varied environment, being, for instance, subject to movement with their surrounding structures, which implies a physical strain, and being also liable to variations in the chemical constitution of the surrounding media. One must bear in mind that the lymph of the central nervous system (i.e. the cerebral spinal fluid) is maintained with an extraordinary constancy of chemical constitution—which is in marked contrast to the lymph of the rest of the body. One indirect evidence of the greater specialization of the tissue within the central nervous system is that the purely nervous elements have lost their capacity for repair after gross injury, being in this respect unique. If the fibres within the central nervous system are more specialized along the line of development of nervous tissue, impulses would be generated and propagated along them with less expenditure of energy than in peripheral nerves.

Effective stimuli may, therefore, be much weaker than any studied by laboratory technique in the peripheral nerve fibre. For this there are two reasons: first, the threshold would naturally be lower as a result of the greater specialization, and, secondly, an impulse coming in by an afferent nerve would produce the most suitable kind of stimulus for the generation of further impulses. We are probably justified, therefore, in conceiving of the central nervous system as containing a network of nerve cells that would keep impulses going almost indefinitely, provided an infinitesimal amount of energy were supplied by the surrounding fluids in the form of whatever may be the "fuel" for a nervous excitation.

This network scheme implies a practical continuity of conduction between unit neurones in the grey matter—in effect a physiological syncytium. Mayer has shewn that an impulse in the detached margin of the bell of the medusa Cassiopeia can go on for weeks. These nerve cells do, of course, form a morphological syncytium. The prevailing view among physiologists at present is rather in favour of a functional discontinuity between neurones that exists in virtue of synapses or similar regions of decrement. Whether there are such blocks or not cannot be proven with present technique. Post mortem staining shews a lack of continuity between adjacent axonal and dendritic ramifications, but it is notorious that the staining of dead and fixed tissues does not necessarily shew all the conditions that may have been present during life: it is only coagulated protein that is stained. There may well be a continuity during life between axones and dendrites in the form of protoplasmic strands that shrivel and retract under fixation or, perhaps, remain unstainable (I have observed an interesting example of this nature when working with vital stains on the central nervous system.[1] With all ordinary post mortem staining methods "pyknosis"—that is a degeneration of nuclear material in which it is concentrated and clumped together in a shrunken mass—appears to involve the entire nucleus, so that there is a clean gap left between the cytoplasm and the apparent remains of the nucleus. Vital stains shewed, however, a nucleus remaining under these circumstances at its normal size, the pyknotic material being evidently only a portion of the total nucleus). Degeneration experiments demonstrate merely that neurones are units from a nutritive standpoint. We must remember that there is a selective distribution of impulses in the nervous system of medusa, although it is a syncytium. Some factor must, therefore, exist which controls this

[1] "Experimental Pathology of the Central Nervous System studied with Vital Azo Dyes", *Psychiatric Bulletin*, January 1917.

distribution, and yet is not to be correlated with anything we can recognize as demonstrable structure. Even if regions of decrement exist in the vertebrate central nervous system they must be less effective than current theories demand, else single stimuli entering by one nerve could not affect practically the entire central nervous system, as they are certainly capable of doing. For instance, in the decerebrate animal a loud sound will increase the reflex responses of practically all the existent central nervous system: this one volley of impulses seems to spread its influence to all the neurones already active. (We shall later have to consider the phenomena of still greater facilitation of impulse-spread that occurs with strychnine poisoning.)

Assuming, then, that the central nervous system is capable of propagating an impulse practically indefinitely, how are we to envisage the paths taken by impulses entering by one or few sensory nerves and eventually producing a volley of impulses in only one or a few motor nerves? If the central nervous system works like a telephone exchange, then there will be specific connections made, the reflex will depend on the integrity of these connections, and vicarious function will be impossible. Such a correlation of structure and function is certainly present in the afferent, and in the efferent, paths but not, as we have seen, in the central connecting and redistributing system. If the simple reflex schema of single afferent, connector, and effector neurones existed, there would be a rigid correlation of structure and function. It is recognized, however, that the connector elements are multiple and complicated. In this complication something must appear that is non-mechanical in its mode of functioning. If we have a system whose function is dependent on the relationship of parts, *qua* relationship, rather than on the sum total of the functions of the parts, then we would have a system that is non-mechanical and satisfies the conditions. Relationships are things that are understood psychologically, they are abstractions, patterns. For their representation material units are necessary, but no one given set of units. For instance, the relationship of three points makes a triangle, but any three points will do (provided they are not in a straight line). In a machine, parts may have to be arranged triangularly but they can only be of certain size, of certain material, and in certain absolute positions, or the machine will not work. So it is in the material world until we come to the atom. Within it, apparently, relationships, *qua* relationships, are what count. The hypothesis I would now advance is that the functions of the central nervous system are to be understood as the product of relationships of points of excitation rather than of the excitation of specific points.

This view is not new but was—unwittingly I believe—put forward by Loeb[1]. Somewhat elaborated—for Loeb's is a sketchy outline—his argument as to the non-localizability of cerebral processes is as follows. Assuming that the residues of past sensory experience of different orders (visual, auditory, etc.) are stored up in specific centres [which has yet to be proved], where is the perception "rose" localized? "Rose," we must remember, is a composite; it is made up of visual impressions, of colour and shape and surface lustre, of olfactory, tactile and probably of motor sensations as well. If we include its name there are in addition auditory and motor verbal elements. In other words, very many centres take part in the formation of the percept. Therefore, says Loeb, it is not localized in any one place but consists of associations of different areas. He does not carry the argument further, but we may do so. Analysed down to its simplest elements, there is not one component of "rose" that does not exist in other percepts as well. "Rose" is, therefore, a relationship existing between these elements. Anatomically, as psychologically, the percept is a composite having its individuality in the proportions and arrangements of its parts. It follows that physiologically, as psychologically, all that is necessary for the excitation of the percept is the establishment of sufficient, localized excitations to form the proportions, relations, or pattern "rose". The anatomical representation we will call "design", rather than pattern, in order to avoid confusion.

Now, if the specificity of the perception lies in the relationship of the cells, or areas, stimulated, it would seem that, so long as this relationship is expressed, there need be no specificity of particular units involved in establishing the relationship. If many elements contribute to the design, the elimination of one or of a few of them will not abolish the design. Three points are essential in forming a triangle, beyond the three any number of points along the lines joining the angular points merely intensifies the design. This explains why injuries to the brain—unless extensive—may produce no loss of function. The function of the cellular units is relational, not mechanical.

[1] *Comparative Physiology of the Brain and Psychology*, chap. XVII.

Vicarious function also follows from this scheme. If part of a design is cut out, the design itself may still be left: for example, if one corner of a triangle, or small arc of a circle, be excised, the design remains triangular or circular. Let us revert to the example of the rose. Suppose the visual areas are destroyed, while other parts of the brain remain intact. The smell or the spoken word will still arouse the perception, as we know from clinical experience; the only inevitable loss is that the perception can no longer be activated by light rays proceeding from the rose. The tactile, kinaesthetic, olfactory and auditory centres can still be co-ordinated in the design "rose".

It is easiest to think of these designs in two dimensional figures. As a matter of fact, they must be at least three dimensional and often, if not always, four dimensional. That time is a factor is obvious when one thinks of the perception of rhythm, so consideration of the time element in cerebral designs may pass with this mention. Its occurrence at the spinal level is not so immediately obvious. The phenomena of summation of stimuli in the scratch reflex, however, would shew that this element must be present at the lower level as well. Other examples could be given, but this is the most striking one, for, as Sherrington has pointed out, no single stimulus, no matter how powerful, will elicit the scratch reflex. There must be some repetition: that is to say the complex of excited neurones which produces this peculiar series of movements must contain a temporal as well as a spatial order of excitation.

The first objection that is likely to arise against this theory is that perceptions are obviously complicated and that the stimuli for spinal reactions are not necessarily so, so that, although the theory might hold for the cerebral cortex, it is not necessarily applicable to the spinal cord. Yet we must remember that Sherrington has shewn that the stimuli for spinal reflexes are often obviously qualitative, i.e. perceptual, in character. One recalls as well the phenomena of local signature, the effect of the previous position of the limb, and so on. But, even if we were without these data, we should have to arrive at the conclusion that "centres" in the spinal cord are composed of previously separated units, on the basis of embryological evidence. The areas of stimulation and the muscles of response represent coalescing and overlapping primitive segments. Each receiving neurone in the cord is probably connected equally with a number of segments and can, therefore, function equally well in the constellation of different stimuli and reflex discharges. Once the central nervous system of the higher vertebrate type is evolved, there is no specificity of function on the part of single neurones (except in the anterior horn cells which are part of the efferent nerves); the specificity lies rather, I should say, in the relation of one stimulated neurone to other stimulated neurones.

The effective stimulus for a specific muscular movement of a reflex order is, therefore, the excitement of a number of neurones in a specific relationship. This design is determined by the immaterial patterns I have been discussing all along. How this is done I do not know, for it is the fundamental mystery. Could I explain it, I could probably explain as well why one dividing ovum turns into a rabbit and another into a man. All I have tried to do is to analyse the phenomena, so that the mysterious action of the immaterial on the material can be narrowed down to one point of contact, so far as the central nervous system is concerned. Fundamentally we are dealing here with a problem in philosophy. In this connection one remark may not be out of place. If the modern view as to the nature of the nervous impulse as an electrical phenomenon be sound, the selection of what neurones are going to be excited must depend on some changes of an electrical order. I should like to point out that this is no more mysterious than the passage of an electron from one orbit to another in the atom with absolute instantaneity, as is, apparently, demanded by the quantum theory. If one can conceive of this, it ought to be possible as well to conceive of patterns determining anatomical designs.

If patterns are made of image functions and liminal images, how are we to imagine the corresponding anatomical designs? A liminal image would be an incomplete design and an image function a completed one. If impulses can be propagated freely throughout the central nervous system, many neurones may be—in the waking state—in a condition of sub-excitability. This might correspond, in part at least, to Head's vigilance. If certain of these are excited still further, the "suggestion" of a design may occur. This is then a liminal image; when the necessary, added neurones are stimulated so as to complete the design unequivocally an image function would appear. The following diagrams would represent this in a two-dimensional arrangement.

It should be noted that (1), which is a liminal image for an octagon or circle, is already the completed design for the image function which would be represented by the square design. These four points in the same rectangular relationship are still present in (2), (3) and (4), but the square has now lost its individuality. This is a graphic illustration of the way in which larger patterns are built: when the various units are thoroughly integrated, previously distinct elements lose their individuality. In absorbing its initial parts into the new unitary whole, the pattern or the design abolishes the original characteristics peculiar to the unit just as a brick loses its individuality when built into a wall.

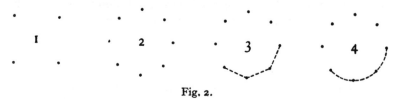

Fig. 2.

An important point to bear in mind is that, according to this theory, impulses are constantly wandering about the central nervous system. If any design is to be established so as to gain dominance over all the other potential designs (i.e., liminal images), it must be formed rapidly. The more highly complicated is any reaction, the more widely distributed is its design, and the greater will be the necessity for speed of conduction. On this basis, the variations of vigilance produced by physical agencies may be explained. For instance, we may consider the case of chloroform which knocks out progressively the most complicated co-ordinations of function. It probably does not—directly at least—change the ionic concentration in the electrolytes but is more likely to affect the insulating membrane. Exposed to its normal environmental influences, the change in the membrane is from permeability to impermeability. If it suffers any other change, the latter, or its specific repair phase, will interfere with the delicate re-adjustment, which is its normal function. This can be easily understood from the analogy with injured or calloused skin, which is no longer capable of transmitting delicate tactile discrimination. If the membrane be injured in this way, a slowing of impulses will result, for reasons discussed above. The effect of this would be to reduce the range of impulses that must act in concert for widespread co-ordinations. Competent reflexes are, therefore, reduced more and more to a segmental distribution. In a further stage of the poisoning, reflexes of the voluntary system disappear altogether, although visceral ones, which are known to have a slower reaction time may persist. If administration of the poison be pushed still further, these too are abolished and, all activity of the nervous systems having disappeared, the organism ceases to be an integrated unit and death results.

Essential to this theory is the notion that the central nervous system prior to the reception of some special stimulation is not wholly passive. Impulses are wandering around from neurone to neurone, although external evidence of the activity is lacking until some group (design) becomes predominantly active. There are probably two sources for these vagrant impulses, the viscera and the afferent nerves of the voluntary nervous system. This is concluded from two types of evidence. A sudden sound or almost any other stimulus will increase the activity of the reflexes in a decerebrate animal, which must mean that the general excitability of the central nervous system has been augmented in consequence of the entrance into it of more stimuli from the periphery. A complementary kind of evidence is derived from a study of spinal shock, which we must now consider.

CHAPTER XVIII

SPINAL SHOCK

WHEN the spinal cord is cut completely through, so that connection between the head centres and those in the cord is broken, temporary symptoms appear which are known as spinal shock. All the voluntary musculature innervated by the isolated portion of the spinal cord is flaccid and stimulation to this part of the body produces no externally observable results. This affects the lower part of the cord which is still attached to the brain as well, but here the effects are nothing like so marked. Within the detached cord, moreover, the effects are more prominent in the headward than in the tailward extremity. The earlier view was that the effects of shock were merely those of trauma transmitted mechanically throughout the mutilated cord. Sherrington has shewn, however, that this cannot be the major factor, because a second cut further distal does not produce anything like the same degree of shock as it would have to do were the effects those of gross mechanical injury. The blood pressure falls, but is soon re-established together with its reflexes, unless the cord be actually destroyed. The functions which are least affected are those which may exist if the cord be entirely done away with, i.e. those of the involuntary nervous system. Wasting occurs in the flaccid muscles, but this is not nearly so marked in animals which are exercised with reflex experiments. The effect is deepest in monkeys and in man, in whom, of course, the cerebral hemispheres are more highly developed than in other species. On the other hand, shock ensuing from removal of the cerebral hemispheres is not so severe as when the pons is also cut off. During recovery, the visceral reflexes first re-appear, then the nociceptive reflexes, and, finally, those associated with the function of locomotion.

As an explanation of these phenomena, Sherrington favours the theory of "isolation dystrophy". "The withdrawal from the isolated cord of influences it is wont to receive from centres further headward may induce an alteration of a trophic character in spinal cells." If we assume that there be such a trophic change in the spinal cells, how are we to imagine their recovery from this injury if their customary receipt of impulses from the higher centres is done away with for good? Apparently, the exercise of such functions, as the isolated cord is capable of performing, serves to rehabilitate the activity of the spinal cells and to negative the trophic change. This is an assumption of use perfecting function, which in this case carries with it the implication of physical regeneration as well. This assumption is, in effect, the one fundamental and vital claim that I am making when I discuss physiological processes in terms of "patterns".

The explanation I would give for the phenomena of spinal shock is as follows. The impulses in any part of the cord which give it "vigilance" come from all the neurones in the central nervous system directly or indirectly, but particularly from those which are concerned with the functions that are maintained constantly in waking life, as well as from the cells active in visceral reflexes, which go on even during sleep. The latter group are small in bulk compared to the former, which include the wide-spread postural system. So long as we are awake, some posture is being maintained, and practically every posture involves reflexes that operate throughout the whole length of the spinal cord and brain stem. When a large number of cells are isolated from the spinal cord that has previously been receiving the bulk of its activating impulses from them, the remainder have not a sufficient number of autochthonous stimuli to keep the local machine running. The deficit may, however, be somewhat reduced by the reception of stimuli from the organs which are connected with the isolated cord, the chief of which is, of course, the skin. These will wake up the segmental reflexes first, since these have a short distribution in the spinal cord. As these short reflexes become more active, their surplus excitation will wander further and further afield, so that designs with a wider distribution may be activated. Finally, a large number of designs will be capable of excitation and a new equilibrium will be established which gives the behaviour of "the spinal animal". The effects are chiefly at the oral end of the isolated cord, because the cells in this region are the ones that have been getting a larger proportion of their impulses from the head region. The visceral functions are least affected, because so many of the ganglion cells concerned in their reflexes lie outside the central system, and the latter receives a comparatively small proportion of its normal impulses from that source. The profound effect of spinal shock on monkeys and on man is to be ascribed to the fact that in these species a larger proportion of the total number of nerve cells lies in the head region. The greater effects produced by section, that cuts the cord off from the pons, than from a section which separates merely the cerebral hemispheres, is at first a little puzzling, because there are so vastly many more nerve cells in the hemispheres than in the pons. It must be remembered, however, that the normal chronic excitement of the spinal cord comes more from the large postural reflexes than from the cerebral hemispheres whose influences are always slight (although highly important) and usually episodic. But the postural reflexes are maintained throughout the waking state. Now, postural tone seems to be a function operating very largely through mid-brain structures, so that when the connection of these with the spinal cord is severed the large designs corresponding with the postural patterns necessarily lapse. It is interesting, in this connection, to note that during sleep, when posture is no longer present, the threshold for spinal reflexes is much higher; i.e. a condition analogous to that of spinal shock exists temporarily. The early re-appearance of the nociceptive reflexes follows from the above considerations: they are largely—or at least primitively and primarily—segmental responses so that designs extending for a short distance only in the spinal cord from the point of entrance of the afferent impulses may serve to activate them. The corollary of this is that the locomotory reflexes whose designs have a wide distribution are the last to appear, and, indeed, they never return in their completed forms, but only as comparatively simple isolated elements.

Sherrington comes close to expressing this view. He mentions that sometimes extensor rigidity occurs, and then remarks: " It is not difficult to see how this may come about. Some incidental circumstance determining the preponderance of some passive attitude of the limbs [pattern accidentally activated] during the early days succeeding the lesion may, by its influence on the inter-action of the recovering spinal arcs, impress an unwanted reflex habit upon the limbs ".

At this point, a comment on the meaning of spinal reflexes should be made. In the intact animal, the "spinal" patterns are well absorbed and integrated into cerebral spinal functions. The animal becomes "spinal" only when primitive patterns become isolated and function alone. According to my view, the patterns of the intact animal cannot be lost (being immaterial and, therefore, indestructible), but simply have not the physical structure through which to express themselves. The spinal animal is a new creature: the primitive patterns which can operate through the surviving structures, and so establish the reaction type known as "spinal animal", once existed independently (phylogenetically). But this was in an animal that had not yet developed the specialized structures, which the modern mutilated animal has. The very essence of pathological reactions is here exemplified: Primitive patterns control specialized structures which ought to be controlled by specialized, i.e. more complicated and more highly integrated, patterns.

There remains to be considered one symptom of spinal shock, the flaccidity of the muscles. This means that they are not merely not contracting but that they have no tone. Tone is a peculiar state in a muscle that is not only a readiness to contract; it is a non-progressive tension. If the tendon of a muscle which is not actively contracting be cut, the muscle shortens, apparently in response to this tension. But tone also disappears under inhibition. In the next chapter we shall see that inhibition of a reflex means a de-activation of the central nervous system design corresponding to the reflex. The normal sub-excitability of the neurones is then lacking.

Tone in muscle is curiously like attention in the mental field. There is the same readiness to respond, when either is present, and this can be inhibited in each case under analogous circumstances. Attention, we concluded, is due to the preliminary excitation of orientation patterns as liminal images, with a reciprocal inhibition of other patterns. Physiologically, we represent liminal images as sub-excited designs. In the waking state, postural patterns distribute impulses throughout the central nervous system as liminal images—i.e. sub-excited designs for postural reactions. Tone may then be regarded as postural designs activated only to a sub-liminal level. (This is not to be confused with Sherrington's "postural tone" and the "shortening reaction".) When the patterns for posture are no longer capable of expression, as in the isolated cord, tone naturally disappears. Hence the flaccidity of the voluntary muscles in spinal shock. (Tone is also diminished during sleep, when posture is absent.)

CHAPTER XIX

INHIBITION

ANOTHER series of phenomena, that demand translation into terms of patterns and designs, are those subsumed under the title of inhibition. This topic is peculiarly pertinent to the general enquiry of this book, because, under the name of repression, the process of inhibition has become as important in contemporary psychopathology as it is in physiology. Unless the phenomena labelled inhibition are really of different natures, the same general formulae ought to apply in the mental and bodily fields alike.

In studying attention the conclusion was reached that the activation of one pattern was apt to involve the temporary inactivity of others. Sherrington has shewn that the same principle is still more marked in spinal reflexes, a principle incorporated in the term "reciprocal innervation". This inactivity appears when, under certain circumstances, a given reflex can be liberated only by a stimulus much stronger than is normally required. Thus the obvious kind of inhibition is detected. On the other hand, a reaction may be liberated by a stimulus of normal strength but exhibit an unwonted intensity; a pre-existent inhibition is then inferred to have been in operation and to have curtailed the activity of the response. The question naturally arises as to whether these two inhibitions are really the same or not.

Let us begin with the first. A good example appears with the flexion reflexes in opposite hind legs: if the reflex be elicited in one of the legs, it is extremely difficult to obtain it in the other coincidentally. This, however, is associated with another reaction, namely crossed extension, which normally tends to appear with flexion; that is, if the right hind leg be flexed the left hind leg will be extended. The complete flexion response is, therefore, not limited to one limb, but tends to include an extension in the opposed one. If the opposed one be now stimulated appropriately for the production of flexion, two incompatible reflexes are stimulated at the same moment, because obviously the leg cannot be flexed and extended at the same instant. The intact animal of course can contract the flexor and extensor muscles simultaneously, as is, indeed, necessary when any graded discriminative response is to be made. But in the spinal animal these combined contractions do not occur under ordinary circumstances, so that, when one group of muscles is in active contraction, the antagonists are inhibited, and it is easily shewn that the inhibition is a product of something that goes on within the central nervous system. We might say that when one set of neurones is active another set is not merely inactive but is relatively incapable of being excited, that is, some positive effect is being exerted. That there may be positive inhibitory stimuli is further suggested by the existence of the specific inhibitory nerves. For instance, there are separate inhibitory nerve fibres running to the abductor muscle of the claw in the crayfish. In the highest mammals a similar differentiation of function seems to occur with the vagus nerve, stimulation of which leads to glandular inhibition, slows the heart beat and also, curiously enough, increases the demarcation current in heart muscle, which is opposite to the effect produced by stimulating other nerves running to muscles.

We have already in Chapter XVI considered the principal mechanistic theories that have been put forward to account for inhibition within the central nervous system, having found none of them satisfactory. The synapse theory or that demanding the secretion of a specific inhibitory substance is essentially tautological. The Keith Lucas and Adrian theory of a region of decrement, which is blocked with more impulses that it can carry, has also been criticized on technical grounds, so that we may now proceed to examine the availability of the pattern and design hypothesis as an explanation of the phenomena presented under the heading of inhibition.

If a pattern is expressed by the distribution of impulses in certain groups of neurones, this implies a relative or absolute quiescence in other, neighbouring ones.[1] There must be a con-

---

[1] Beritoff ("On the Fundamental Processes in the Cortex, etc.", *Brain*, vol. XLVII, p. 109) speaks of a possibly similar view put forward by Pavlov in a Russian publication: "...inhibition arises around the focus of excitation. It is said that this occurs in accordance with the special law of contrast of nervous activity. This is a rather peculiar law, according to which the excitation produces inhibition around itself".

trast in the degree of excitation of the neurones before a design can appear. On the background of diffusely circulating impulses, a design might be established by super-excitability in some neurones and sub-excitability in others. This makes contrast an essential feature of formation of designs. It can be understood, perhaps, by a simple analogy. A graphic design may be represented as well with black ink on white paper as with white chalk on a blackboard. Intrinsic, therefore, to the very concept of anatomical designs is the notion of inhibition as well as excitation. This would account for the inactivity of muscles whose function is opposed to that of the reacting ones; but why are they so difficult to stimulate?

The group of neurones controlling the contraction of even one muscle must be complicated, as is evident when one recalls the phylogeny of the mammalian muscle and nerve structures. It is, therefore, probable that whenever a muscle contracts (except perhaps during fibrillary twitching) some design is operating. Our study of attention shewed that before a pattern is stimulable it must be present as liminal images, and that concentration of attention means the reduction or abolition of inappropriate liminal images. We may assume that the same thing happens in the central nervous system. When the diffusely circulating impulses fall into groups, the designs corresponding to antagonistic reactions are in a state of sub-normal excitability. That does not mean necessarily that the separate neurones are inexcitable individually, but that any stimulus penetrating this particular part of the nervous network is not distributed by a pattern. The impulses will wander in a random manner throughout the quiescent area, and will not activate a specific series of neurones simultaneously, as they should do to form a design. The necessary constellation of cells could only be activated synchronously if the stimulus were strong enough to flood the entire area with impulses. This is the same thing as saying that the reaction has a very high threshold. It is seen, then, that the quiescent area is in a state comparable to that of the whole spinal cord when it is suffering from shock. There is a vacuum so to speak that has first to be filled before the normal pressure is reached, the normal pressure corresponding to the threshold. A further addition of pressure—of nervous impulses—will produce the surplus that appears as discharge.

The modification of inhibition by higher centres follows from the pattern theory. New integrations are new patterns, this being the very difference between combination and mixture. When under cerebral control, antagonistic muscles may contract simultaneously, and there may then be patterns which are not $\frac{\text{flexion}}{\text{extension}} = \frac{1}{0}$ as with spinal reflexes but $\frac{\text{flexion}}{\text{extension}} = \frac{3}{2}$, or some other similar proportion. If we were to regard the coincidental contraction of flexors and extensors as algebraic sums of opposed reflexes, i.e. as mere mixtures, then we might be forced to conclude that there was an inhibition of the spinal inhibition allowing the two reactions to take place at the same time. But this is an assumption which denies the actual integration of the spinal reflexes into larger patterns. As a matter of fact, it is the sort of thing that occurs in the learning period of new movements, before the integration of the new patterns is complete, a phenomenon well illustrated in playing unfamiliar games. With direct voluntary control the discriminative movement is slow, clumsy, *and* fatiguing. It is, therefore, probably wrong to speak of inhibition by higher centres when higher integrations are working normally: the spinal reflexes are not inhibited but really have disappeared as such, being incorporated into larger, alternative patterns.

On the other hand, there are phenomena appearing, when the integrity of higher centres is interfered with, which do look as if they represented an escape from inhibition. There are violent reactions of the spinal reflexes, spread of contractions from one muscle group to others (which may be totally absent in the intact animal), and, perhaps the product of these two, the appearance of reflexes that cannot be elicited in the intact animal. (An example of this is the so-called Babinski phenomenon in man: when the pyramidal tracts are injured the application of a noxious stimulus to the sole of the foot produces an upward bending of the toe, which cannot be voluntarily imitated. It is probably to be regarded as part of a total flexion reflex.) Analogous phenomena occur in the psychological field, when instinctive reactions appear on the lapse or weakening of consciousness, and unconsciously motivated behaviour is seen, which is absolutely foreign to the normal personality. Can these be correlated in terms of patterns and neuronic designs?

According to my theory, when a design is completed, it produces the complete response. Every pattern, then, represents an all-or-none reaction. The activities of the "higher" centres do not, however, shew explosive activity but graded response. This, I suggest, is due to there being innumerable patterns operating through the higher centres, each one corresponding to a slight difference in response. An automatic telephone exchange gives a highly discriminative reaction to a specific stimulus, yet that response is of the all-or-none order. The bell is rung with equal violence in all cases, or not at all. The spinal reflex is like a connection made with a whole local exchange, so that every bell is rung. In the spinal condition, discrimination is made only between the different type reflexes, the exchange is called, so to speak, rather than just one number in it. The mechanism ringing one bell is not inhibiting the mechanism ringing the whole exchange: they are different mechanisms.

There are limits to this analogy, however. It seems to hold where the higher centres are expressing well-integrated patterns. For instance, the more complicated reaction of flexion + crossed extension + inhibition of crossed flexion is a later pattern phylogenetically than is simple flexion, yet, when spinal shock has passed away in a dog, it almost always appears, and in decerebrate animals is invariable. Here we are dealing, however, with a pattern that is still very old and thoroughly integrated. The same uniformity of response is notoriously absent when the more highly integrated pattern is of recent development and when it is not associated with an anatomic specialization. A new pattern is unstable relative to older ones. If unstable, it will operate sometimes and sometimes fail. In the latter case, the more primitive, wholesale kind of reaction will appear; in the former, it does not, its place being taken by a more discriminative one. This certainly looks like inhibition coming and going and, when a strong sudden stimulus elicits the old indiscriminate reaction, the conclusion is almost inevitable, that inhibition has been overcome.

According to my view, however, the discriminative and the non-discriminative reactions are alternative ones, rather than that the non-discriminative one is inhibited by a positive opposing influence exerted by the discriminative reaction. The problem is, then, to formulate the conditions under which one rather than the other pattern operates.

If the structures in the central nervous system necessary for the reactions are both intact, two factors will operate to decide the choice. The first is a physical one. If the initial excitement activates neurones common to both designs, spatial proximity will decide which is to be activated first, provided both patterns enjoy the same degree of integration. For instance, the knee jerk in man, or the flexion reflex, is apt to follow immediately on a sudden application of an appropriate stimulus and co-ordinate movements to succeed it, only when the attendant image functions have activated the designs for the more discriminative behaviour. When the discriminative design is largely cortical and the non-discriminative is sub-cortical or spinal, it is obvious that this difference of distance to be travelled by the spreading impulses might be considerable. Moreover, cortical designs are probably more complicated. These two factors would predispose the cortical reactions to fatigue or poisoning earlier than those of the lower neurones. On the other hand, practice may so integrate the more discriminative patterns as to give them dominance. For example, the primitive reaction to a blow threatening the face is blinking of the eyes, retreat and throwing up the arms, so as to ward off the blow. A boxer gradually substitutes discriminative responses: before the substitution is complete, there is a point where both are equally automatic. At this stage, fatigue will give a preference to the simpler type of reaction.

All conscious reactions are more recently acquired than "instinctive" ones, the latter, therefore, tend to predominate when the stimulus is sudden or the subject is fatigued, or they tend to come first with the conscious ones following later. One may be startled by a sudden noise and then react discriminatively to it; or, if the subject be exhausted, the same stimulus may throw him into a settled panic. The greater frequency of phobias and night terrors in children than in adults is probably to be traced to the fact that conscious discriminative reactions are still so recent as to be highly unstable integrations: in consequence any stimulus suggesting danger produces a primitive danger reaction, which then absorbs all the energies of the organism, the impoverished consciousness being too weak to deal discriminatively with the situation.

But, if conscious reactions are always less well integrated than instinctive ones, and if they involve in their expression more extensive neuronic excitations than instinctive ones (as they very likely may), why are they ever reactions of choice? The answer is, perhaps, to be derived from the psychology of attention and of meaning. Every stimulus breaks into an equilibrium consisting of patterns either actually in operation or represented by liminal images. This equilibrium may contain elements in it pertinent more for one reaction than for another. A simple example is the flexed limb giving extension on stimulation, while the extended limb responds to the same stimulation with flexion. My interpretation of this is that liminal images of the stepping reflex are present (meaning). Somewhat similar results were obtained by Sherrington and Sowton, who found that weak faradic stimulation to the internal saphenous nerve gave extension instead of flexion, *if postural tone were present*. It is this same principle, probably, which makes extension the dominant reaction in decerebrate rigidity. Posture, being continuous and not episodic, is present before the stimulus is applied. This posture, being one of standing, includes extension at least as liminal images. The threshold for extension is, therefore, low, although it is not so primitive a reflex as is flexion. The latter having no favouring background has lost its position as reaction of choice.

Consciousness and personality are highly complicated patterns, or systems of patterns, involving integrations built of simpler patterns ranging from the reflex and instinctive levels upwards. When consciousness is operating, therefore, liminal images are present for all the patterns relevant to the stimulus towards which the organism may be oriented. Discriminative response then occurs not in virtue of a superior integration of the discriminative pattern, but because the pattern is already potentially active.

We must now consider the spread and the bizarre reactions which occur when "control" functions lapse. Whether we are speaking of mental functions in a person with normal interests, or the wandering of impulses in a healthy central nervous system, one reaction tends to set up more images or image functions. The normal fate of these is to activate more patterns. If higher integrations are potentially active (as in the alert mind or intact central nervous system), the secondary reactions will be coordinate and adaptive to the situation to which the organism is oriented. If, however, orientation is lost—lapse of consciousness or discontinuity between lower and higher centres—it is the more primitive patterns only which can operate. This accounts for the spread and bizarre reactions. They have not been repressed so long as the higher integrations were operating: they were alternative reactions that had lapsed, for generations perhaps, if physiological processes, for a few minutes perhaps, if mental processes. In the well-integrated personality, as in the healthy central nervous system, subliminations or highly integrated patterns are completely dominant; and during waking life are superior to all the other reactions. That is, theoretically they should be. Practically, as we well know, personality is rarely so well integrated. The more primitive patterns have many opportunities to spring into being, particularly when consciousness lapses during sleep or drowsiness.[1] What is the nature of the processes by which these primitive patterns are relegated to the unconscious?

We have concluded that there is no inhibition, properly speaking, with perfectly and automatically working higher patterns. But, with the less efficient integrations, there is a real possibility of choice between primitive and discriminative responses. Moreover, if the integrations be of a highly complicated order, it is easy to see how the liminal images of two patterns might, many of them, co-exist. They would come into conflict only when the completed patterns demanded use of the same element for opposite purposes. Neurologically, this would mean that movements which are carried out by anatomically widely separated muscles and which only accidentally coincide in co-ordinations of the whole organism, would not tend to arouse liminal images that were mutually incompatible. For example, leg reflexes and movements of the vocal cords can proceed together. These would come into conflict only when the leg movements were so violent and continued as to result in difficult breathing. The respiratory reflexes are, of course, integrated with laryngeal ones. Many visceral reflexes are similarly capable of performing their functions in practically complete independence of voluntary reflexes, the latter affecting the former only by the slow influence of metabolic change (accumulation of waste products and exhaustion of oxygen supply, etc., during prolonged muscular contraction). Other anatomically separate muscles may at times function separately and again come into conflict. Fine co-ordinate movements of the fingers can

---

[1] Were the integrations of personality perfect, there would be no variations of reaction unless new patterns were set up by unique experience that produced new combinations. With the perfection of reaction patterns achieved during advancing years, personality becomes better integrated, but a heavy price is paid: imagination fails and intellectual sterility ensues.

co-exist with leg movements; for instance, a man can button up his coat while he is walking. But finger movements and arm movements are inevitably integrated together. Hence, if the leg movements are part of a complex co-ordination involving extensive and accurate arm movements, the latter will conflict with the finger movements. One could not jump a stream and button his coat in mid-air at the first trial, because the arms are here essential for balance. Movements which can be carried out simultaneously and in response to different stimuli are *dissociated* functions. So far as the physiology of voluntary muscles is concerned, the possibilities of dissociated function are limited on account of the inevitable overlapping of patterns in bodies that perform innumerable co-ordinated movements with a small number of parts.

The situation is different in the mental field. Images or ideas not issuing in conduct can theoretically co-exist and continue to flourish quite dissociated, so long as they do not tend to use the same pattern, or system of patterns, for incompatible ends. Psychologically, the expression of a pattern is its emergence into consciousness, which is the analogue of expression of physiological patterns in movement. (How this comes about will be considered in a later publication.) Consciousness cannot, at the same moment, harbour two incompatible ideas or images more successfully than a limb can flex and extend at the same time. The reason for this is that consciousness is, so to speak, the organ for the expression of programmes of activity, just as a limb is the organ for the expression of a single action. The ideas or images concerned with totally different programmes of activity can co-exist, therefore, so long as they do not both tend to come into consciousness. Thus unconscious mental life can exist that is totally at variance with conscious mental activities, and there will be no conflict between the two systems until the unconscious tends to become conscious. At this point, a choice of reaction, a conflict, appears; and, with this, that inhibition of the unconscious patterns which we know as repression.

Inhibition in the physiological field we have reduced to the partial and preliminary activity of the dominating pattern in the form of liminal images. Can repression be reduced to the same general terms? I think it can, although a full explanation will only be possible when the genesis of personality and consciousness have been discussed in a later work. We can say now that

personality is an integration of interests. The nature of a per
sonality depends on the interests that are combined to form it.
Interests operate as liminal images determining attention, meaning,
etc. Whether a given reaction pattern will be integrated with
consciousness or not, depends, then, on the presence of liminal
images suitable for absorption of the pattern or incompatible
therewith. If the latter, no integration of consciousness with the
pattern ensues: in other words, it is repressed. This is the same
formula as for the physiological process of inhibition.

But the fate of the patterns inhibited may be different according
as they are physiological or psychological. In my scheme a physiological design involves blank spaces—a network of neurones
that are inactive. A stimulus penetrating this inert region is not
distributive so as to form a design, since it has no pattern to guide
it. The disturbance which débouches into this vacuum, so to
speak, has its origin outside the central nervous system and, on
cessation of the stimulus, ceases to exist. This is suppression,
annihilation, not repression. The unconscious processes that fail
to unite with consciousness have, however, originated within the
central nervous system and are not extinguished, just because they
fail to achieve a particular integration with other patterns. On the
contrary, this tends rather to their perpetuation. What quiets the
disturbance in the central nervous system seems to be an efferent
discharge—a summation effect endures only until the reaction
takes place. Similarly, penetration of unconscious processes into
consciousness seems to put an end to their activity.[1] Failure of an
unconscious process to enter consciousness tends, then, rather
towards its prolongation. The effect of the inhibition of mental
processes is their repression, whereas that of physiological processes is suppression.

This conclusion would seem to be at variance with our main
thesis that mental and physiological processes follow the same
general laws. It must be borne in mind, however, that with every
increase in complication of patterns, as integrations become more
and more elaborate, changes in behaviour of the patterns emerge.
As noted in the "Laws of Patterns" III (b), the more simple and
fundamental are patterns, the more repetitions are there needed to
establish them. Physiological patterns are of this order, so much
so that generations are needed for their integration. Sherrington

[1] See *The Psychology of Emotion*, p. 553.

has succeeded in obtaining a graded reflex response in a spinal animal by carefully adjusting the strengths of stimuli for opposed reactions. Sufficient repetition of this procedure would in time, according to theory, establish the pattern for the reactions that are normally inhibited. Such artificial conditions are, of course, incapable of repetition during a sufficient number of generations for their integration. The inhibited reaction has, therefore, no chance for continued existence on the physiological level. At the mental level, however, even a single coincidence of reactions is sufficient to integrate them. Hence patterns for unconscious ideas may be formed, and perpetuated so long as they remain unconscious. This difference of behaviour between mental and physiological patterns under inhibition is, therefore, inevitable.

Finally, a word should be said as to the possible biological nature of the so-called inhibitory process, which we have concluded to be a negative rather than a positive affair; that is, the stimulus for a reaction that is inhibited simply falls on non-reacting tissue. Blank spaces are just as important as reacting areas in the neuronic network, if designs are to exist; and, from the neurological stand-point, that a cell does not respond is enough. But, biologically, one cannot cease to wonder why this should be. In considering the evolution of mental processes, it may be well enough to begin at a reflex level where patterns already exist, but, from an evolutionary standpoint their first appearance is a problem. What could make a nerve cell specialized for the propagation of impulses in-sensitive to stimuli, except such grave injury to the whole structure as would mean abolition of function for a long time? I naturally cannot give any final answer to this question, but should like to put forward a suggestion.

No matter what view may be taken of the physico-chemical nature of nerve impulse, it is clear that it involves some kind of energy transfer. Energy is liberated in one part of the fibre and passed on to the next portion. This energy must somehow be made good again, if the nerve is to go on performing its function. The energy discharge must be followed by some kind of re-charge. If it be katabolic, there must be an anabolic phase following it. If it be a physical disintegration, there must be a consecutive stage of re-integration. This secondary phase, in terms of patterns, is what I would call the repair reaction. It has two inevitable characteristics: it must be specific in that it makes good a specific loss and its direction of reaction must be opposed to that of the primary disturbance. Nerve fibre has then two specific and dia-metrically opposed properties: liberation or propagation of im-pulses and a reconstitution of the substance destroyed in generation of the impulse. One is just as important as the other. If one assumes—which may be a large assumption—that the repair function can exist dissociated from impulse production, then we would have two processes, opposite in nature, which by com-bining in varying proportions could account for neurones being active or passive to stimulation. These are the only conditions necessary for the development of designs within the central nervous system network. The existence of a refractory period followed by a stage of super-normal activity (in weakly acid media) is strongly in favour of this view. If the impulse depends on a breaking down of a specific structure or material, the more there is of this substance the greater will be the impulse. If the refractory period represents the phase of repair, its continued over-activity would produce the surplus giving the subsequent super-excitability. The effects of certain drugs can be expressed fruitfully in terms of their influence on the repair reaction. For instance, strychnine may perhaps facilitate repair, while anaesthetics retard it.

CHAPTER XX

THE EFFECTS OF STRYCHNINE ON
THE CENTRAL NERVOUS SYSTEM

STRYCHNINE is said to abolish reflex inhibition and convert it into excitation (analogous symptoms are produced by the toxin of tetanus). This would seem to be equivalent to a statement that strychnine abolishes designs and allows impulses to spread diffusely and lawlessly: that is, a purely physical agency annihilates an immaterial guiding principle, the pattern. If this be so, it would seem to indicate that our formulations are at fault, that the pattern is a product of structure, since it is abolished by injury to the structure. Further, it seems to suggest that synapses are essential to the structure allegedly underlying the pattern. Peripheral nerve is little affected by strychnine, if at all, and its action seems to lie in the grey matter where synapses are present. This view is supported, moreover, by the failure of strychnine to convert inhibition into excitation, where inhibition operates peripherally and not centrally; for example, when there are special inhibitory nerves. Again, the drug is said to have little effect on the nervous system of invertebrates, where the network of nerves is a syncytium, the "non-synaptic" type of nervous system. These are serious difficulties.

When in strychnine poisoning a single stimulus such as a loud sound will throw all the voluntary muscles of the body into tetanic contractions, agonists and antagonists alike, it looks as if impulses were spreading diffusely and rapidly throughout the whole central nervous system. On the other hand, cerebral functions are unaffected. The latter would indicate that only the lower or spinal type of cells are involved. Consonant with this view is the fact that sensory thresholds are lowered and this action has been shewn to be peripheral and not cerebral, for local injection of strychnine will raise the acuity of vision in one eye and not in the other.

Lowered threshold in my terminology is a heightened activity of liminal images. Let us suppose that the effect of strychnine is simply to increase the irritability of neurones. This could occur, theoretically, by the difference of potential between the electrolytes within and without the nerve fibre being raised, or by the speeding up of the permeation and reconstitution processes in the membrane. What would now be the effect of patterns operating through such a structure?

In the first place, such a nervous system, although it would respond more readily than a normal one, would still need external stimuli to set off any reaction. This is shewn to be true. Cutting the afferent roots of the spinal nerves abolishes strychnine convulsions. Secondly, when a given reflex was called forth, the threshold being low, the stimulus would provide excess energy which would go towards the activation of integrated patterns and thus the impulse would spread more widely than in the normal organism. (This question of the fate of the surplus of the stimulus energy over and above the threshold requirement is a matter to be discussed in a subsequent publication under the headings of gradation of response and fatigue.) Thirdly, the super-excitability of the neurones would tend to elevate liminal images into image functions and new reflexes would be excited *via* these image functions, rather than by externally derived impulses. Fourthly, these new reflexes would again set up stimuli of a proprioceptive order, and it is to these that we might trace the apparently anomalous effect of inhibition being turned into excitation.

Evidence from various sources seems to indicate that any reflex tends to limit itself by setting up image functions of opposed reactions.[1] When a muscle contracts it stretches its antagonist, i.e. it increases a tension already existent in virtue of tone. This tension provides a proprioceptive stimulus, a duplication and, therefore, an augmentation of the liminal images which are the basis of tone. In the normal central nervous system, the initial excitations constituting the existent tone are of such a low grade that they are easily abolished and, when gone, provide the negative background for a design. If under strychnine these excitations are more lively, they will be harder to abolish. Reciprocal innervation will, accordingly, not be so complete. When an agonist contracts, the tone of its antagonist will not be abolished: it will therefore be ready to contract. A proprioceptive stimulus will

---

[1] This is a matter to be discussed in detail under the heading of fatigue in a later publication.

effect this. Ordinarily the proprioceptive stimulus does this slowly, merely inhibiting the after-discharge and preventing any given reflex from going on indefinitely. Under strychnine, however, this counteraction is so quick as to occur at the same time as the initial contraction. Both agonist and antagonist contract at the same time. It is not, then, a question of inhibition being turned into excitation, but, rather, of inhibition never having been complete and of counter-reactions that should appear only after withdrawal of the stimulus occurring contemporaneously.

There is some experimental support for this view. Cushny[1] says: "Baglioni has shewn that a single stimulus is not sufficient to cause complete tetanus, but that the movement induced by the first shock leads to secondary stimuli arising from the joint and tendons which are moved; the arrival of these secondary stimuli in the cord maintains its activity and the muscles remain contracted until the cord is fatigued and refuses to react to the persistent stimuli from the periphery". Sherrington has performed experiments shewing the mechanism more in detail. The toxin of tetanus has an action on the central nervous system similar to that of strychnine, but is slower and more gradual in its action. It is, therefore, possible to analyse its effects. He says: "In the gradual progress of the condition I have several times found the hamstring nerve produce slight inhibition of the extensor, if the initial posture taken at the knee be extension, and yet produce distinct excitation of the extensor if the initial posture taken at the knee be flexion". Here we have a stage, then, in which the over activity of the extensor design neurones is not sufficient for any proprioceptive stimuli to be adequate alone, although, when the extensor muscles and tendons are already stretched by the flexed posture, the first slight increment of tension in the extensors is sufficient to produce a proprioceptive stimulus that will cross the threshold. A somewhat similar bit of evidence comes from Baglioni's demonstration (as quoted by Sherrington) that the prolongation of reflexed contractions, which is characteristic of mild strychnine poisoning, is due to excitations of proprioceptive reflexes, secondary to contractions set up by exteroceptive stimuli.

Essentially the same principle may be invoked to account for the effects of strychnine on breathing reflexes. Haldane[2] says: "The analogy between the Hering-Breuer stimuli transmitted

---

[1] *The Action of Drugs*, p. 272.   [2] *Respiration*, 1922, p. 10.

through the vagi and what Sherrington has named the 'proprio-ceptive' stimuli participating in reflex or voluntary movements of the limb is evident... ". These stimuli are those proceeding from inflation or deflation of the lungs. "It was evident from these experiments, and from the marked slowing and deepening of breathing after the vagi are cut, that distension of the lung stimulates the nerve endings of the vagi in the lungs in such a way as to terminate inspiration and initiate expiration, while deflation of the lungs produces a corresponding stimulus acting so as to terminate expiration and initiate inspiration. Thus inspiration seems to be the cause of expiration, and expiration of inspiration. Hering described this as the 'self-regulation' of breathing." In breathing, then, there are, as in walking, alternative tensions determining the reciprocating contractions of agonist and antagonist muscles. If liminal images be exalted by strychnine, a lesser degree of inflation ought to stimulate deflation, and so produce more rapid shallow breathing in the poisoned animal. If the administration of the drug were continued, the liminal images would become image functions and a beginning inflation lead at once to deflation. Such effects are observed, for Cushny says: "The respiration is quickened by small quantities of strychnine, especially when the centre is depressed by the previous administration of a narcotic... a reversal of the respiratory reflexes is sometimes seen after large doses in animals and it is analogous to that described in the inhibitory reflexes of the spinal cord". During convulsions, of course, breathing is apt to be arrested as a result of the violent contractions of the trunk muscles.

It is now easy to see why strychnine should not affect the cerebral functions unfavourably. Its action is merely to facilitate the activation of liminal images and image functions; but these are excited under the guidance of patterns. Cerebral designs may, therefore, appear with greater facility, but they will still be normal designs. This is because cerebral functions are not reflexes, that is, they are not responses to external stimuli but only to internal ones, and the latter follow a patterned distribution. The potential activity of the sub-excited neurones may be greatly heightened, what are normally fully quiescent areas may provide liminal images, but, failing further stimulation, a liminal image does not become an image function. And this stimulation can never come so long as the impulses are guided solely by patterns. In the cord, however, under exactly the same conditions of excitability, the liminal image neurones receive stimuli from the periphery, *via* the proprioceptives, and at once produce image functions. Cerebral activities do not produce externalized muscular contractions, which inevitably throw back into the cerebrum an echo of proprioceptive stimuli; these afferent impulses débouche into the spinal cord, not into the cerebral cortex.

These conclusions form a corollary to the earlier generalization about the necessity of speed of conduction for the existence of widespread co-ordinations. Specialization of nerve structures facilitate conduction and *ipso facto* makes possible new integrations, new patterns that are dependent on the factor of speedy conduction. A pattern is correlated, then, not only with a specific distribution of impulses, but also with a rate of distribution. Its nature can be changed by altering either factor. If the rate of spread of impulses in a complicated integration be speeded up, muscular contractions that ought to be successive will become synchronous. That is, agonists and antagonists, which ought to contract alternately, will contract together: a new and pathological reaction is thus formed, and this is the symptom tetanus.

CHAPTER XXI

BIOLOGICAL PATTERNS
PREFORMISM AND EPIGENESIS

So far, in speaking of the relation of patterns to structure, I have often treated the latter as if the central nervous system were a mass of neurones forming a network not differentiated into specialized tracts and centres. This is obviously not the case. There is a specialization of structure that is correlated with certain fundamental functions and the correlation involves two things: great efficiency in the operation of function and dependence of function on the existence of structure. The latter is shewn most plainly with the great conduction tracts, for instance, the posterior columns of the spinal cord are essential for *rapid* co-ordination, as is shewn in the disease of locomotor ataxia in which degeneration occurs in these columns with resultant inco-ordination as a symptom of the disease. (The occasional brilliant results achieved by re-education of patients suffering from this disease shew that the patterns can work through collateral paths, or, at least, that roughly equivalent patterns can do so.) This rigid correlation is confined to the conduction tracts, but localization of function in various centres is also an unquestioned fact. For instance, the reflexes involved in respiration depend for their continued function on comparatively small areas in the medulla and pons remaining intact; similarly, a large number of postural reflexes seem to operate through structures confined to the neighbourhood of the red nucleus. In these cases, however, the boundaries of the centres cannot be fixed with accuracy, and considerable injury may be done to the centre without permanent loss of the functions pertaining thereto. Finally, we observe functions that seem to operate through quite extended regions of the central nervous system, where the use of the term "centre" is justified only by analogy, and where vicarious function is notorious. Most of the functions of the cerebral cortex are of this order and the mass reflexes of the spinal cord should, perhaps, be classified here as well. The latter certainly shew an extraordinary degree of recoverability after an acute attack of anterior poliomyelitis or disseminated sclerosis. The problem presented by these discrepancies in correlation between structure and function must now be considered, a matter involving some rather fundamental biological principles.

This introduces the question of the interdependence of structure and function. It is usually assumed that structure is fundamental and primary, function being the inevitable expression of the physical and chemical properties of structure. There is, however, a mass of evidence pointing in the other direction, which is commonly ignored. Teleology is taboo with most biologists, although —which is quite amusing—a mechanist is apt to be dissatisfied with any hypothesis which does not explain purposeful reactions in materialistic terms. That is, he admits the phenomenon: it is, in fact, his absorbing problem; but he is happy only when he can call it by some other name than "purpose". If his explanation does not fit in with the phenomena which others would label as purpose, he doubts its validity.

If we begin, however, with the data which refuse to fit themselves into the mechanistic theory, it may be possible, perhaps, to elaborate an alternative view. This would involve a complete reversal in theory and make function responsible, ultimately, for structure.

The practice of function undoubtedly improves function, and there are many examples, in other than the neurological field, of this being associated with a perfecting of structure. The growth of muscle with exercise is, of course, notorious. Better examples appear, however, in bones, because there the change is graphic and striking. In the healing of a fracture, a mass of bone called callus cements the fragments together. This has no regular architecture, as has the normal bone with strands of mineralized tissue running in the direction of the lines of stress in the bone. Such architecture will appear in the callus only when the limb is used. This is function determining structure. It occurs, however, not merely with bony scar tissue. When, as a result of accident, disease, or habitual change of posture, the direction or distribution of stress in a bone is altered, its architecture will change, adapting the structure to the new mechanical conditions. This is known as Wolff's Law. Many a child has curved legs until it stands and walks on them, when they straighten out. If the shin-bone be broken in three parts and clumsily reset so that the ridge in front is not in line with those above and below, the prominence will in the course of months or years gradually shift round into line.

In these cases, structure is certainly being modified—specialized —in response to function. Moreover, in the case of the change in callus following use, there is a differentiation of tissue, which is like that observable in the phylogenetic differentiation of specialized organs. Another example will illustrate what I mean by this. Herbivorous animals have a much longer digestive tube than have carnivora, but such a lengthening may be produced in one individual by change of diet. Babák[1] reports that the intestine of tadpoles will vary enormously in length and thickness, according as they are fed on animal or vegetable food, being nearly twice as great in the latter case. To derive the ultimate origin of specialized organs in general from such functional influences involves, of course, the assumption of the inheritance of acquired characteristics, which is inconsistent with Darwinism as now interpreted, although not inconsistent with what Darwin himself claimed. If the continued use of the structure leads to the growth of a specific part of the organ, as in bone, this would seem to be analogous to, or identical with, the phenomenon in the psychological sphere of practice leading to further integration of a pattern. In the anatomical material the integration is demonstrated morphologically. If the pattern theory have universal biological applicability, it should be possible to explain evolution of structure in the same general terms as one uses in explaining the evolution of mental patterns.

This application of the theory can only be considered with great brevity. We must first see to what extent the idea of patterns is implicit in current theories of development. In so far as pattern means specific appearance and arrangement of elements, it is, of course, recognized by all biologists, and, indeed, is incorporated in the laymen's phrase "like breeds like". But, when it comes to a matter of identifying the agencies which produce this uniformity, there is marked divergence of view. Three positions assumed by different schools must be considered.

The first is the predeterministic, or preformist, school. Its view is that the adult organism is a mosaic of small elements, each of which develops in relative independence of the others or of external factors, and functional unity is achieved only when the

[1] *Arch. Entwick. Mech.* vol. XXI, 1906.

mosaic is formed. These elements are the pre-determinants of Weissmann or the genes of contemporary geneticists. They are physico-chemical entities, and individual development depends on their physico-chemical properties alone. The phenomena of chromosomal development lead the present day exponents of this view to assume that every cell in the body inherits the entire equipment of genes of the fertilized egg. The physico-chemical properties of the genes lead inevitably to growth and development of the various organs. This is the materialistic point of view in its most unequivocal form.

In opposition to this school stand the advocates of epigenesis and vitalism, who assert that the peculiar differentiation of each individual organ is the result of external factors. It is pointed out that, if development depends merely on the physico-chemical properties of elements within the egg, then there would be no differentiation of parts. So long as the genes are dividing, so as to duplicate and multiply themselves, and are exposed to no influence inoperative in the fertilized ovum, differentiation is impossible. One cell makes two similar ones, these make four, and so on, but, under the conditions stated, all new cells will be like their parents and the individual will only be a mass of identical cells. This objection is so obvious that the pre-determinists pay lip service to other factors in such phrases as "regional differences in the egg". But these extra factors thus admitted play no rôle in further specula-tion. The final theory is summed up in Morgan's phrase that develop-ment is the product of "the collective action of the genes". These writers stoutly affirm that the house is made of bricks, but refuse to consider the work of the architect and even of the contractor.

Whence comes the regulating factor which causes the differ-ential development of the various units? Two answers are given, the one metaphysical and the other physiological.

The vitalists or neo-vitalists admit frankly that no solution of a materialistic nature is possible, and remove discussion from the physico-chemical field by the assumption of an *entelechy*, a meta-physical principle, which is the essence and regulating principle of each organism. This entelechy seems not to be a law of nature, but something supernatural. That the guiding principle is im-material, I too claim, but, if I understand the neo-vitalists aright, they take no account of the influences that make the entelechy (which I should call the individual pattern). It is more of a given, pre-existent and pre-ordained, and wholly metaphysical entity, whereas my pattern is more of a law of nature—not a law that is merely a generalization of phenomena observed in the past and a descriptive affair, but rather a law in the sense of a regulating agency. The difference may be represented in an analogy with two deities. There is the God of the first chapter of Genesis and there is Mother Carey in *The Water Babies* who "makes things make themselves". Pattern psychology, or pattern biology, is a study of how things make themselves.

On the other hand, there are those biologists who stress the physiological aspects of development. The claims and arguments of Charles M. Child[1] may be taken as exemplifying this school. He too uses the word pattern and makes it cover the processes of development as well as the behaviour of the adult organism. His pattern, however, is a descriptive term for a sequence of arrangement of events, rather than for a guiding principle. He admits—even postulates—the existence of material units, or "potentialities", in the developing protoplasm, and accounts for the differentiation of the various regions and structures as the product of a differential development, instituted by environmental factors. The egg is subjected to different degrees of stimulation in its different parts from differences of temperature, light, gravity, oxygen or nutritive supply, etc. Such differences establish different rates of metabolism or of living, and thus a "physiological gradient" is formed. This gradient means differential rates of growth—a purely quantitative factor at the outset—which leads to different qualitative results. For instance, an egg may derive nourishment from an attachment at one pole. Oxidation and, therefore, growth become greater at the opposite pole; growth then proceeds along the line joining the two poles, and thus an axis of the organism is formed. Physiological gradients are demonstrated by differences of oxygen and carbon dioxide exchange, differences in permeability and of susceptibility to poisons, and by differences of electrical potential. The last is most important. The part that is chemically most active, that is living at the highest rate, seems to dominate the more lethargic area. This, Child and his co-workers have demonstrated with a wealth of experiments. The dominance determines struc-

---

[1] Child has written three books in elaboration of his theories: *Senescence and Rejuvenation*, 1915; *The Origin and Development of the Nervous System*, 1921; *Physiological Foundations of Behaviour*, 1924. The last gives an ample summary of his views.

212 BIOLOGICAL PATTERNS PT II

tural differentiation and, if the communication be blocked, or the gradient abolished, the tissue specialisation ceases or regresses. Impulses of some kind seem to pass along the gradient, and Child considers them to be of an electrical order. Conduction, then, the fundamentally "nervous" phenomenon, is a factor in embryological development. It is not difficult to see how Child arrived at the conclusion that there is something in common between growth behaviour and organismic behaviour! His work is based on a large amount of apparently well-controlled experimentation, and is, of course, carried into the detail of many gradients, appearing in the course of development, and their interrelation. This we cannot go into here.

It would seem to be indisputable that Child has discovered an important embryological and physiological principle in the gradient. He has emphasized and made more specific the interdependence of one part of the body on others; he has shewn that co-ordination is a much more fundamental and universal function than is an anatomically developed nervous system. He has furnished a more adequate scheme of development than that of the preformists, but he cannot be said to have eliminated the mystery. Even he has to fall back on "potentialities of the protoplasm", that cannot be accounted for on either a pre-deterministic or on a physiological basis. One example—out of many—may suffice to shew this. The egg of the alga *Fucus* develops its physiological gradient—its axiate structure—from the differential action of light. But, he admits, if kept from differential exposure, it will in time develop its gradients spontaneously. This is due, he says, to a potentiality of the protoplasm which is transmitted; the effect of earlier differential exposure to light has affected protoplasm, so as to give it a tendency towards development of a physiological gradient. In the reconstruction of the complicated developments in higher forms of life it is, of course, necessary to assume such transmitted gradients very often. Now, this kind of potentiality in the protoplasm is just the very element which materialistic biologists are trying to eliminate, whether they be pre-determinists or epigeneticists. Child speaks of it—like Semon—as a protoplasmic memory. Peculiar comfort seems to be derived from tacking the adjective "protoplasmic" to a mental entity: it seems to enable the mechanist to think that he is getting along without the assumption of an immaterial factor.

We cannot, then, accept the physiological gradient as the sole cause of differential development, if the gradient be looked upon merely as the blind working of physico-chemical causes and effects, producing differentiation of structure simply by changes of rate in these physico-chemical processes. What Child's experiments do demonstrate, however, is that specialization of structure is dependent on co-ordination of growth; that organs, or parts of the body, do not attain their adult morphology in isolation, but only in relation to growth and function elsewhere. In other words, it is the pattern of the organism which determines the specialization of the part. That Child has tried to base this pattern on a purely materialistic factor and failed does not detract from his proof of the existence of the pattern. It was already indicated by a large series of biological observations, which his experiments have amplified and organized into a sound descriptive formula: specialization of structure is dependent on integration of the part with the whole. The converse he has shewn to be equally true: disintegration, or physiological isolation of the part, leads to de-differentiation of the part or, as we would say in our more general terms, it leads to a regression that is in this case morphological.

The axiate pattern of development in the alga *Fucus* seems to operate more quickly if the egg be exposed to a differential light stimulus, but will appear spontaneously in time. This would seem to be an example of a pattern containing a liminal image of differential light exposure (or of the metabolic effects thereof), but capable of producing the differential-activity element as an image function.

It must be borne in mind that patterns in the mental field are modes of response to stimulation which gradually become more perfect. They are, therefore, dependent for their appearance on previous activity either within the organism or external to it—they do not come out of the blue; and they have their evolutionary history, their gradual integration. In other words, they are not sudden and special creations: they do not appear like Athena springing full armed from the head of Zeus. If the same kind of patterns operate in morphological development and evolution, we must look for proof of them not in the phenomena which appear with apparently inevitable spontaneity, but in those processes where integration is not yet perfected, where there is obvious dependence on stimulation from without, i.e. the liminal image phase of integration. If development or evolution presented only a series of easily separable stages, or of forms that appear with an inevitable spontaneity, the vitalistic theories would be the best. It is the imperfect development and the transitional stages that shew patterns in the process of development, which shew that patterns are integrations of evolving functions, rather than functions the expressions of pre-existent, fore-ordained, metaphysical agencies.

CHAPTER XXII

BIOLOGICAL PATTERNS
THE EVOLUTION OF SPECIALIZED TISSUE

IN reconstructing any scheme of evolution, one has to begin somewhere. Any substance having the characteristics by which we recognize life is probably already differentiated and has had its earlier evolution. But, for our present purpose—which is not the origin of life—we may begin with protoplasm. Protoplasm is a substance, or substances, that is identified by functions, not by chemical constitution, for the latter varies in different species. It can digest suitable foreign matter and build it into more protoplasm. It exchanges oxygen and carbon dioxide with the environmental medium. It has mobility, the whole mass or parts of it being extensible or retractable. It can reproduce itself, be it only by the simple process of one bit splitting off and growing by itself. If injured locally, the part that has been "killed" may be digested or cast off, and new protoplasm formed to take its place; it thus maintains its identity in a changing environment. A stimulus given to one part may affect distant regions; conductivity is thus present. Its surface tends always to be differentiated physico-chemically from the interior. It has thus the functions of digestion, circulation, respiration, contractility, reproduction, protection and conductivity, without having any morphologically visible stomach, blood vessels, lungs, muscles, gonads, skin or nerves. Such morphological differentiations as may be observed in simple protoplasm seem to be evanescent. The structure which is at this moment pseudopod and motile is in the next withdrawn and has lost its individuality.

If the evolutionary hypothesis be accepted, we have to account for the appearance and progress of two sets of phenomena. First, the above-mentioned functions become more or less identified with permanently differentiated structures, and second, the functions themselves are vastly improved. The final result is such a close relation between the specialization of the organ and the correlated function, that the latter seems to be merely the blind and inevitable expression of the physico-chemical nature of the former.

According to the Darwinian hypothesis (in its contemporary form), structures appear by chance and are assumed to perpetuate themselves in subsequent generations. If the morphological variation be favourable to the maintenance of the life of the individual, those who inherit the variation are favoured in the struggle for existence: they survive and the undifferentiated individuals all die. According to de Vries' mutation theory, the original modifications are not so slight as Darwin assumed, but chance is still invoked.

On the other hand, Lamarck considered the variations to be the product of environmental influences. This is a more satisfactory hypothesis, since it eliminates pure chance, but the preponderance of experimental evidence has been definitely against characters thus acquired being transmitted to the next generation. The Lamarckian hypothesis is, therefore, in disrepute. Biologists on the whole have preferred to accept the theory that involves pure chance—a scientific unhappiness—and includes a further mystery, for it has yet to be shewn how or why variations once established should carry with them the capacity of transmissibility to offspring. This mystery I cannot dispel; on the contrary, I would try to magnify it as but one manifestation of the laws of patterns, which are a codification of the mysteries of life, be they psychological or morphological. In other words, the mystery of mental life is the same as the mystery of evolution, and it is not incapable of formulation in terms of a law or laws. Moreover, the pattern hypothesis does not involve such a scientifically unpalatable assumption as special creation, or the special creations, which the chance variations of the Darwinian theory imply. We do not need to assume peculiar forms or origins of energy unknown to the physicist, but merely the regulation of the application of energy within the organism by those immaterial agencies, the patterns. And this kind of regulation is something appearing in the phenomena upon which the quantum theory is based, in the growth and working of our bodies and in the operation of our minds.

Anything like a detailed explanation of the phenomena of evolution in terms of the pattern theory would be out of place in this book. I can only suggest its applicability at certain points.

If one begins, as all biologists do, with undifferentiated protoplasm, we find that the simplest form of life, which we can recognize as such, has a certain individuality. It is capable of maintaining itself relatively unchanged in a changing environment.
Capable of, and presenting, a large series of physico-chemical
reactions, these are so integrated that their sum total maintains a
unity which we define as life. The most complicated syntheses or
associations of chemical substances artificially brought together
fail to achieve this unity and so are, biologically speaking, dead.
That is to say, physico-chemical laws alone will account adequately
for all the behaviour observed in the synthesis. When life begins,
some factor that defies physico-chemical analysis has appeared.
This factor is then, by definition, an immaterial one, for matter
is what behaves wholly in confirmation with physico-chemical
laws. The presence of this immaterial factor is evidence of a
pattern, or patterns, being already present in the simplest protoplasm observed or conceived. The origin of this first integrating
principle, i.e., the origin of life, is not our quest, which is, rather,
its subsequent development. I am merely trying to emphasize
that, in accounting for evolution, we are entitled to take for granted
the previous appearance and continued existence of this unifying,
integrating principle.

We commence, then, with a conception of a primordial protoplasm, which shews the series of functions, or in other words, a
series of physico-chemical reactions. The peculiarity of this series
is that its elements are integrated together. In the material world
reactions go on until the supply of an element necessary for a
chemical combination is exhausted, or until an equilibrium of
electrical forces is achieved. At this point, the reaction ceases and
is begun again only when some outside agency provides more of
the element necessary for the combination, or upsets the equilibrium. In an integrated system of reactions, when one of them
comes to an end, for either of the above-mentioned physico-
chemical reasons, the others, somehow or other, reconstitute the
conditions which made the reaction possible. If it be a chemical
combination, more fuel is automatically supplied; if it be an
electrical affair, differences of potential are again set up. Thus is
the unity of the organism maintained, which is life. The peculiarity of living matter can be reduced to one property, differen-
tiating it from any known artificial associations of non-living

matter. When any reaction takes place in the organism, the condition of physico-chemical instability, which gave rise to it, is reproduced. This is true, moreover, for each and every reaction entering into that total integration which constitutes the organism. In the morphological field, this reconstitution takes the form of replacement of worn or injured parts and is known as repair. I shall, therefore, name this peculiar property or reaction of matter from its most obvious manifestation, but I wish to make clear that "repair" may be quite an invisible process, and includes such subtle events as the re-establishment of electrical potential or polarization.

It has just been argued that living tissue is alive in virtue of its capacity to maintain itself, i.e. an integration of its various functions exists, and this integration implies an equilibrium. Disturbance of the equilibrium is the stimulus for the reaction, and this reaction will go on until the equilibrium is re-established. In a simple physico-chemical system such as an oxidation, for example, the intensity of the reaction gradually diminishes as the supply of oxygen (or of the material to be oxidized) is exhausted and the reaction comes to rest. The duration of the reaction is dependent on the supply of fuel, and, unless more fuel be supplied, it will cease. Now, in a living integrated system, no reaction is as simple as this. The supply of fuel or oxygen (assuming the reaction to be an oxidation) is not passive but active, because the equilibrium is upset so soon as depletion of the material for some reaction begins. It is not like a furnace with so much coal in it that will burn until it is exhausted, but rather like a furnace plus a stoker who keeps putting coal in. When any reaction of protoplasm is in progress, it does not occur in isolation and unrelated to the other parts or functions of the protoplasm. The very fact of integration implies that there will be subsidiary reactions set up to restore the equilibrium and having the effect of perpetuating the central reaction, by, for example, providing oxygen or fuel or both. From this it follows that any reaction in protoplasm is going to proceed, until its disproportionate development disturbs the equilibrium which gives the system its unity. Living reactions come, therefore, to an end not by a gradual diminution as equilibrium is established, but only in virtue of the counter-reactions set up when a dis-equilibrium is brought about.

If we turn now to the repair reaction, we can see an interesting consequence of this inevitable behaviour in an integrated system.

Some material is exhausted in the performance of some function and reconstitution of this begins. The protoplasm turns its energies—I am using the term in its physical and not in any metaphysical sense—to the reproduction of this material. This repair is one of the reactions of the living tissue, and, of course, there is a specific repair process to compensate for every specific depletion there may be with every specific function. The repair reaction will go on, as other reactions do, until a dis-equilibrium is established. The reactions to compensate for this in turn, i.e. to restore equilibrium, have their thresholds, and up to the threshold point the repair reaction will proceed. That is to say, not only will the actual quantitative loss be made good, but a surplus will be produced.

In a tissue with a delicately adjusted equilibrium such as a nerve fibre the surplus is not long maintained, but we do find in a nerve a period of super-excitability following the refractory period, and it is to this that a successful summation of stimuli in a decremental region is ascribed. A nerve fibre is isolated in a medium of nearly constant chemical constitution. Its equilibrium can, therefore, be very finely adjusted in proportion to the specialization of its functions, which are reduced to conduction and reconstitution of the physico-chemical structure broken down in the propagation of the impulse. In primitive protoplasm, it having many functions and being exposed to a changing environment, the equilibrium must range between fairly wide limits. Were it not so, it could not adapt itself to its changing environment. From this it follows that the threshold for the re-establishment of equilibrium will be high when a repair process is in action; in fact, the repair itself will tend to establish a new equilibrium in this labile integration. When, therefore, any specific function is performed, the compensatory repair will tend to produce a surplus of whatever physico-chemical structure is destroyed in the production of the original reaction. Function will accordingly cause a growth of the specialized physico-chemical structure necessary to that function.

Over-repair is responsible for specialized growth.

From this it is easy to understand why exercise of a specialized tissue leads to its further development in the individual organism. A muscle contracts and thereby loses or injures some special chemical substance, or breaks down some special electrical polarizations. This is more than made good by repair, so that this structure is now bigger and will give a stronger contraction the next time it is stimulated. (In rhythmic contractions repair probably itself furnishes the stimulus for the next contraction, as it rebuilds to the point of instability.) The bigger the muscle and the stronger the contraction the more extensive will the destruction and repair processes be: the muscle grows cumulatively, its limits of size being determined by the equilibrium of the body as a whole, operating largely, perhaps, through metabolism. Similarly in bone, repeated pressure or tension leads to deposition of mineral salts just at those points where the force is applied, where protoplasm is destroyed in its function of passive resistance, and where inert solids are, therefore, laid down. Hence the apparently marvellous architecture of bones, which is merely the inevitable expression in form of the great central mystery of the repair process which "makes things make themselves", and which is, as we have seen, integral to life itself as a phenomenon of maintained individuality in a changing environment.

This, however, is merely the process of further specialization in an individual organism of a tissue already specialized. The original specialization must be accounted for, that is to say, evolution must be explained. In primitive protoplasm the exercise of one function will lead to increase of the physico-chemical structure necessary for that function. But such structures are diffused, apparently, throughout the whole organism. This makes true specialization impossible. Suppose, for instance, that a series of specific stimuli excite repeated contractile, or muscle-like reactions; excessive repair will then lead to the protoplasm becoming preponderantly muscular in type and, therefore, losing its individuality as an equally functioned tissue. Three possibilities appear as to the fate of a primitive organism under such conditions. First, it would die, second, the unifying integrating tendency would inhibit excessive over-repair, and, third, the growth of the contractile substance would indirectly excite the growth of other elements in virtue of the general integration which means equilibrium. In none of these conditions will specialization result. This can occur only when conditions are such as to make possible a repetition of similar stimuli and similar responses in one part of the organism throughout successive generations. It will then differentiate and do so indefinitely. What are these conditions likely to be?

The first is rather obvious. The surface and the interior of any mass of protoplasm are subject to different conditions. This means that there will be a differentiation of function between the outside and inside of the mass. For instance, the inside will never participate in pseudopod reactions and chemically its environment will be more constant. Consequently, the inner mass will have a more stable metabolism. While the chemical composition of the periphery may vary with intake of food, and so on, the central mass will have that chemical constitution characteristic of the protoplasm in question. It will then perform different functions. If we were dealing with a non-living combination of substances, this difference would shew itself only in a higher rate for certain reactions at the centre, which would be slower as the periphery was approached and *vice versa*, and no sharp line of demarcation would ever appear. But it is a living system; therefore, whatever region is performing any given function preponderantly will tend to differentiate for that function. The periphery accordingly specializes in the direction of contractility and the early stages of digestion, while the central part specializes for the later stages of digestion— the synthesis of the compounds peculiar to the protoplasm in question. Thus, the nucleus, or rather, nuclear substance, is differentiated and we can speak with perfect accuracy of an organism for the first time.[1] Nucleoplasm is acid, while cytoplasm is basic in its reactions. Between them there must be a neutral zone. It is, in all probability, this boundary zone that becomes the nuclear membrane. Since the central mass of what is now a cell is the unchanging part, it is what maintains the individuality of the cell and so is naturally the vehicle for transmission of inherited specific qualities.

Another point must be borne in mind. The nuclear substance is isolated from the changing environment not only by the cytoplasm but by the nuclear membrane as well. Living in this isolation it is able to specialize still further in a degree impossible for cytoplasm. Further specializations will then be associated with, and integrated with, the nucleoplasm that lives in isolation. No matter what changes may take place in the cytoplasm, the nucleoplasm can go on evolving, developing a more and more delicate

[1] Child has made a similar suggestion as to the origin of the nucleus, deriving it from the difference of conditions at the centre and periphery, but not elaborating the hypothesis further. (*Origin and Development of the Nervous System*, pp. 60, 61.)

chemical specificity. The specificity of the organism will then not only lie in the nucleus but will depend on the integrity of the nucleus, since these later developments are the product of chemical functions that can take place only when the nucleoplasm is insulated. A corollary of this is equally important. Identity of the cell being relegated to the nucleus, the cytoplasm is free to specialize in any direction without imperilling the individuality of the cell.

We now have an organism differentiated into two structures with different functions. One is used in maintaining the identity of the cell and the other establishes contact with the environment, getting food, and protecting the more delicate nuclear substance. If general mobility and motility be essential for the existence of this cell, it is difficult to see how evolution could proceed further, for there could be no constancy of stimulation of one type at any part of a constantly changing body. But if we imagine the organism to be in the medium which brings its food to it, as, for instance, a fluid containing oxygen and food in solution (or the food in drifting particles), then it can do as well attached to some object as moving itself about. Once attached, a differentiation of stimuli and, therefore, localized specialization of function is possible. One part becomes a "foot", will receive no food and no noxious stimuli: it will grow more sticky on its surface and the tissues within will differentiate to withstand the displacing effects of current in the water. The external surface immediately next the attachment will not participate in movement, and so will have constantly two sets of stimuli from within and without acting upon it. This will favour the development of a membrane. If the environment furnished noxious stimuli, mere membrane substance, i.e. neutral material, will be further differentiated, and thus an integument or skin will be formed. We can imagine further changes resulting from this. The basal integument becomes tough and relatively immobile; then the opposite extremity will do most of the moving, put out the pseudopodia and get in the food. As the free pole becomes more motile, the basal extremity will become more digestive, and so on. The organism may then break loose and swim with its pseudopods, now become flagellae. Different organisms have doubtless developed in countless different sequences, but all, perhaps, following this general kind of scheme. That is, once chance allows a repetition of similar stimuli to fall on one part of an organism, that part will differentiate to perform the function appropriate to the repeated stimulus, and this differentiation will of itself lead to greater and greater specialization of stimuli to the other parts of the body, with consequent differentiation in them.

Sherrington[1] makes a great deal of the relationship between axiate development in an animal, with its progression along the line of the axis, and the development of the special sense organs in the anterior end. He points out that the correlation is close between opportunity for frequency of stimulation of any order at any given point in the body and the extent of development of receptors in that region. This is shewn not only in the specialization of different species, but also in the development of the individual, for he cites a number of examples of animals that lose their eyes on assuming a sedentary habit. It is locomotion forward which brings a large number of light stimuli to the head region.

But, it will be at once objected, this is an assumption of evolution in one organism that would have to be well-nigh immortal, if it were to live long enough for all this development. These are changes requiring repetition of stimuli over thousands of years. How was the improved response to a given stimulus transmitted to the offspring, so that it can go on with the evolution? This brings us to growth patterns.

[1] *Integrative Action of the Nervous System*, pp. 323, 324 and 333 seq.

CHAPTER XXIII

GROWTH PATTERNS

THE first of our Laws of Patterns is: "When specific stimuli are applied to an organism synchronously or in immediate succession, each being of sufficient intensity to produce its appropriate reaction, there is a tendency for the reactions to become united together, forming a pattern". Now, when a specific function and its compensatory repair reaction occur, there are successive reactions, which by this law will tend to be integrated together. The first effect will be a lowering of threshold for the repair phase. After a sufficient number of repetitions, the repair reaction will appear with less and less display of the specific function and, therefore, of the destruction which the repair is to make good. Finally, the stimulus may lead over directly to the exhibition of repair. Repair, which is not compensatory for loss, is growth; and when, in the course of embryological development, a stimulus appropriate for a given function seems to call forth the structure which will perform this function, then we have a growth pattern, in which the function in question has become an image function. When the establishment of one structure results in the localization of different functions in other parts of the organism, as, for example, when the fixation at one pole determines mobility at the other, then these functions will in time be integrated into their appropriate growth patterns. Finally, the secondary growth patterns will be integrated with the first, and with one another, so that an integrated system of growth patterns emerges, which guides the development of the organism as a whole.

These patterns will, of course, be gradually developed through countless generations. Let us take the hypothetical example of the sedentary unicellular organism. Its medium is favourable for sedentary life, and, therefore, in many generations attachment to a solid object takes place, until the patterns for the function and structure of attachment are established. It has now become a sessile organism and the various developments at the free pole can begin. These will have their further effects, and so on. It might be urged against this hypothetical reconstruction of specialization in consecutive generations that the same pole would not always be attached. This is quite true, but irrelevant, if the pattern theory be sound. Either the organism when it becomes attached has already differentiated a "foot", or it has not. In the former case, the "foot" will attach itself. In the latter, we are dealing with a cell having undifferentiated protoplasm: any part may attach itself. Now, if the pattern has already begun to be formed, the fact of attachment will be the stimulus for activating this pattern, which can operate from all poles equally well, since the pattern is primary, and the structure results from it secondarily. Indeed, Child has shewn this with his gradient pattern. If the tissue in question has, as he says, the potentiality of gradient in its protoplasm, appropriate stimulation will establish the gradient from the point of application. Moreover, he has shewn that a gradient once established may often be reversed by strong enough stimulation from another point. So it is, from our point of view, a matter of complete indifference for the story of development at what points the organisms may attach themselves in successive generations.

One corollary of this scheme is important to note at this point. The pattern for a specialized function is established first and its structure secondarily. Therefore, functions will be transmitted from generation to generation before the specialized structure appears. Finally, the associated repair reactions will be integrated, and then a "variation" in the morphological sense comes into being. If inheritance is, first of all, of function, it follows in turn that the patterns which are the most easily established—namely mental ones—will be the first and most easily transmitted. This may not amount to the spontaneous reappearance of a new mental reaction; it would rather be a lowered threshold for the reaction. This may account for the ease with which dogs can be taught to retrieve, for instance, which can hardly be the result of selective breeding, for carrying a live bird uninjured is, presumably, not a natural habit in a wild animal of the canine tribe. One might similarly account for the rapid establishment of national types.

Proof is not lacking, however, that acquired physiological reactions may be transmitted as well as mental ones. For the

demonstration of this it is necessary to use organisms that reproduce with great rapidity. Bacteria fulfil this condition. That
the virulence of a micro-organism can be increased by passing it
through a series of susceptible hosts, or diminished by growing it
in artificial cultures, has been a truism of bacteriology ever since
Pasteur's brilliant demonstration thereof.[1] Similarly, Paramoecia
have been bred to live at temperatures originally lethal. The
theory of patterns shews why Lamarckianism is unlikely to be
proved experimentally in the morphological field. Under III (b)
in our laws of patterns it is stated: "The more primitive a reaction,
the more repetitions are needed to establish it as a pattern."
From the standpoint of the adult organism, the growth patterns are
the most primitive elements in its total integration. The number
of repetitions needed to establish changes in growth patterns are
so great as to involve more generations than experiment can
normally compass. To implant a new morphological characteristic in this manner on a mammal would probably require some
thousands of years, but it might possibly be done with some of the
rapidly reproducing lower organisms within the lifetime of a
laboratory devoted to this quest.

A word should now be said as to specificity of inheritance: as
to how it is—in terms of patterns—that "like breeds like". Why
does the fertilized ovum of a dog not produce a rabbit, and why
can a mammalian ovum be fertilized only by a sperm cell from
the same species? It has long been known that the essential

[1] "Law of Patterns" III (b) may account both for epidemics and their sub-
sidence, which are equal mysteries. It says that higher, more adaptive integrations are more quickly established and more unstable. If a pathogenic organism
varies its virulence slowly, the hosts will develop immunity to it pari passu. In
order to have epidemic virulence it must, therefore, assume a heightened virulence with great speed. This implies instability, so virulence will decline again.
According to this view, offending microorganisms may be old friends of the
bacteriologists which assume a high degree of virulence temporarily. Thus, the
bubonic may suddenly become the pneumonic with its 100 per cent. mortality,
and this is followed by a decline of the epidemic. If it were not for the abate-
ment of the virulence the pneumonic plague would inevitably destroy every
human being on the globe in the course of time. According to this view, we need
never fear that mankind will be destroyed by any epidemic. It is its instability
which gives any organism its epidemic virulence and the same instability means
a subsequent loss thereof.

A somewhat analogous phenomenon was pointed out by Darwin. When in
some one species an organ is much more highly developed than in allied species,
that organ then shews a striking variability in size. In my terminology, the
specialized pattern for the enlarged organ is imperfectly integrated, and, being
so, is unstable, sometimes operating and producing the large organ, but at other
times not.

elements in germ cells are nuclear and, apparently, within the nucleus, the chromosomes seem to be the structures that carry inheritance. Of recent years, students of heredity have narrowed down the elements still further to *genes*, which, within the chromosomes, are the final units, transmitting characteristics from generation to generation.

The genes may be summarily disposed of. They have never been seen or detected as such by any physical means. They are merely inferred to exist. In other words, they are a way of talking about the phenomena of heredity, hypothetical units which, when properly arranged, give the formula for a given heredity performance. They are assumed to have a material existence, because many biologists cling to the respectability of materialistic philosophy; but the laws expressed in terms of genes could be equally well put in terms of patterns. In fact a gene formula *is* a pattern.

We must reckon, however, with the fact that specific developments only occur when specific, physically demonstrable, germ cells are brought together and given the proper amount of oxygen, warmth, etc. Manifestly, these material factors are essential. Why the nucleus should become the seat of the specific chemistry of the cell we have already seen; but now we have to deal with the problem as to how it has come about that immaterial growth patterns should be dependent on specific physico-chemical factors for their expression.

Patterns evolve as the result of reactions performed simultaneously or consecutively. So far as we know, any given pattern does not exist before its gradual appearance after repetition of the component reactions. Physico-chemical factors have, therefore, been present in their formation; physical processes are later guided by them; and without matter to work through they would have neither *raison d'être* nor means of expression. In fact, patterns such as we are now discussing are nothing but integrations of physico-chemical processes. In a pattern of sequential processes, one of them is a stimulus for the next, and a specific one at that. The pattern for the development of a dog is a pattern formed during the evolution of an organism with canine protoplasm. The chemical specificity of the nuclear material in canine bodies has been integrated with the growth patterns and has become an essential link in the chain. Similarly, fertilization by a canine sperm cell is an essential stimulus for the initiation of development.

To repeat the analogy used before, there must be a piano and something to hit the keys before piano music can be played; further, the peculiarities of piano music are derived from the mechanical peculiarities of the instrument. But that does not prove that the piano can compose its own music, nor that piano music may have no existence when a piano is not available. Specific chemical substances in the chromosomes are to the development of an individual what the piano is to piano music.

CHAPTER XXIV

BIOLOGICAL PATTERNS
IMAGINAL PROCESSES

SINCE this is not a biological treatise primarily, I can only indicate the nature of the proof that patterns explain, or at least describe, the phenomena of development more adequately than other formulae. It has been said before that proof of the existence of patterns in my sense depends not on the finished, perfected function, but on evidence of the evolution of that function, i.e. of the lack of perfection in the pattern. This is because the finally perfected pattern has its structure so specialized—so adapted for its specific function—that the function lapses if the structure be injured. The function then appears as if it were merely the expression of the physico-chemical properties of the structure. Patterns have three stages: first, liminal images; second, image functions; and third, such unification of the total pattern that separate image functions have lost all their identity. These three stages can be demonstrated over and over again with growth patterns.

Whenever a stimulus is required for the appearance of differentiation of the tissue in any organ, liminal images are still present in the growth pattern. Studies of the physiology of development are full of examples of this: it is constantly being shewn that the development of one organ is the signal—and the necessary stimulus—for the differentiation of another.

The eye of some amphibians is a good example. The first structure to appear is an outpouching of the brain, which grows towards the skin. This is the optic vesicle. When it touches the skin, the latter begins a cycle of changes which eventually produce the lens of the eye. Not only will the skin fail to produce a lens, unless it be touched by the optic vesicle, but, on the other hand, almost any bit of skin will do so when contact with it is achieved, as has been shewn in transplantation experiments. A certain degree of dependence in development on the practice of the final function may be shewn in the myelinization of the optic nerve in mammals according to Held.[1] "In animals which are blind at birth (cats, dogs, etc.), if one eye is kept closed by sewing together the eyelids, the appearance of myelin in the corresponding optic nerve is delayed."

Complete development may depend, curiously enough, not on performance, or stimulation, of the final function but on the presence of a stimulus conditioned with normal development, apparently as the result of mere coincidence. This is shewn in the case of the final development of spermatozoa in mammals with descended testicles. It was long known that animals (or men) with undescended testicles were sterile, but only recently has it been shewn by independent observers[2] that the difficulty is not in any sense mechanical. Spermatozoa apparently only develop and live if subject to variations in temperature such as are inevitable in testes that are carried in a scrotum and, therefore, outside the body. Moore shewed that if the undescended testicle were chilled, it would produce viable spermatozoa, while if the scrotum were insulated from cold, the spermatozoa would not be completely developed. These thermal conditions have nothing whatever to do with the normal function of the gonads, but seem plainly to be an association accidental to the situation in which the descended testicle finds itself. This is a pure example of a conditioned response in the field of organ development.

Regeneration experiments are equally interesting. (Regeneration may be looked on as the renewed or continued operation of growth patterns after the adult morphology has been attained.) The regeneration of legs or of the tail in amphibia is dependent on the nervous system remaining intact. The nerves presumably transmit some stimulus, some representation of the function to which the specialized growth is a response. The influence mediated by the nervous tissue may be a highly specialized one, as is shewn by the phenomena of restitution of eyes in the crayfish. If one eye be removed and the optic ganglion left intact, the eye will regenerate. If, however, the optic ganglion be also removed, a less specialized structure, an antenna, will appear. A most

[1] *Entwickelung des Nervengewebes bei den Wirbelthieren*, 1909, as quoted from Feldman, *Antenatal and Postnatal Child Physiology*.
[2] See Carl R. Moore, *Endocrinology*, July 1924, who gives the literature on the subject. These experiments were performed in his laboratory and also independently by Fukin in Japan.

interesting example of vicarious growth is reported by Wolff and Fischel;[1] they shewed that if the lens of the eye in certain amphibia be removed it will be regenerated from the side of the iris. Their experiments have been amply confirmed, being well controlled histologically, so as to prove that no ectodermal tissue remained at the site of the regeneration. The striking thing about this is that the lens, which is primarily an ectodermal structure, is here produced from a mesodermal tissue. This seems to be an example of that exhibition of liminal images which I have termed the utilization of substitutes.

So much for liminal images in developmental patterns. We have now to consider the phenomena which may be represented as image functions, and as further integrations of patterns in which given image functions lose their identity completely. How an image function may lose its identity is shewn in the mental field with many perceptions that are unified combinations of many elements. A large number of the latter may lose individuality. For instance, the leaves of a book that lies on a table do not enter as such into the conscious perception "book". What is perceived is a plane surface, flat on the top and bottom and curved on the front. Yet one knows that this surface is made up of the edges of hundreds of sheets of paper. The book may lie too far from the observer for this to be confirmed visually, but the remembered images of separable sheets have nevertheless contributed to the making of a complicated pattern which is the perception. In such a case, the separable leaves are images, or image functions, that have lost their individuality. Phonetics furnishes us with an equally good example. The vowel "i" is a diphthong of "ah" and "ee", but how many people can detect these two elements in it?

Now, we must bear in mind that, according to the present scheme of development, there are these stages in the formation of the ontological patterns: one function leads to growth of a specialized structure; this in turn causes specialization of function in another part of the organism, and, eventually, specialized structure there. Exercise of function is then originally present between all successive specializations of structure. As integration proceeds, actual function is less and less necessary; i.e. liminal images tend

---

[1] Gustav Wolff, "Entwickelungsphysiologische Studien. I. Regeneration der Urodelenlinse", *Arch. f. Entwickelungsmech.* I. A. Fischel, "Ueber die Regeneration der Linse", *Anat. Hefte*, XLIV, 1900.

to become image functions. This produces a stage in which one structure apparently follows another directly. Finally, in the chain of growth reactions, certain structural links may be dropped. These are then image functions that have lost their individuality.

The appearance of gill structures in the embryos of mammalia gives a good example of function becoming purely imaginal. The purpose of gills is respiratory. In fish, water containing oxygen is drawn in through the mouth and passed out through the slits between the gills. In the latter are blood vessels with thin walls through which oxygen and carbon dioxide can pass. In mammalian embryos oxygen arrives from the parental circulation through the umbilical veins and carbon dioxide is excreted by way of the umbilical artery. There is, therefore, no respiratory function performed by these "gills". In fact, they are only rudimentary gills, for the clefts are not completed (with the exception of the first), being merely furrows on the neck outside and the pharynx within. Respiration has here become a pure image function and even the gill structures themselves are on the way to do so, for, before they can differentiate as real gills, they merge into other structures of the head, neck and chest.

Each one of the embryonic gill ridges contains a blood vessel, and these vessels develop into various arteries to the head and neck and one of them becomes the arch of the aorta, which is, of course, in the chest. In a fish the heart pumps almost directly into the gill vessels, so it is practically a "neck" region, or would be if the fish could be said to have a neck. The gill region forms the lower part of the head and organs in the neck (the first gill arch forms the lower jaw and the first cleft is the external opening of the ear). Respiratory and cardiac function are, therefore, located in the head and neck region originally, centring in the gills. In the adult the structures subserving these functions are in the chest, but their nerve supply is still from the part of the nervous system supplying the gill region. Hence the vagus—a nerve from the medulla—supplies the heart and lungs, while the diaphragm is innervated by the phrenic, a nerve originating in the upper neck region.

The gill-like structures of the mammalian embryo shew us, then, functions appearing only as image functions in the total developmental patterns. But the structures themselves are incomplete, rudimentary. They pass on into other structures—jaw, ear, larynx, etc.—or disappear altogether. A rudimentary structure, leading to a different step in development, would seem to be a liminal image stimulus for the adult structure. This final structure cannot develop out of undifferentiated cells; it still has to have some specific stimulus, which is the rudimentary gill. It is so rudimentary that it seems to be on the way to disappearing. When it does so—as it may in the next million years—it will have become an image function that has lost its individuality as it has been absorbed into a larger pattern.

Now, there are examples in embryology of just this, of structures that have become image functions. Some of the somites of the head region have suffered this fate. Somites are blocks of mesodermal tissue, occurring serially and establishing segmentation. In the neck and trunk regions of the mammalian embryo they are still well marked, eventually producing the segmented spinal column. In the adult chest the segmental distribution of muscles and nerves that originate in the somites is still plain (the intercostal muscles and nerves). The basal occipital bone of the skull develops from definite somites which usually coalesce, the segmental character being then completely lost in the adult. In most mammalian embryos, however, there is a stage during which the developing basi-occipital bone looks quite like four vertebrae, although this is beginning to be obscured in the human embryo. Sometimes coalescence is incomplete, so that the lowest part of the occiput remains separate, betraying its independent origin. From these occipital somites there migrate the muscles and nerves to the tongue, an organ which in the adult has no segmentation whatever. Here we have structures still acting as liminal images, but beginning to look like image functions. Further forward in the head all direct evidence of somites in the base of the skull is lost in mammalian embryos, but a mass of data from comparative anatomy indicates that the cartiliginous bones which develop there were originally separate. This latent segmentation accounts, however, for the serial arrangement in the brain stem of the nuclei of the nerves to the eye muscles, which appeared originally as muscles belonging to these somites. Instead, therefore, of having one nucleus for all the eye muscles, as one would expect from their unified function, there are three nerves, the III, IV, and VI, which have their nuclei arranged serially. Accordingly, in a mammalian embryo some somite structures have become pure image functions and, moreover, they have lost their identity completely. The bones of the anterior base of the skull, originally a series of somites, develop now as large units. The somites, then, are fused, just as the edges of the leaves in a book are fused in the visual percept "book".

CHAPTER XXV

THE DEVELOPMENT OF
THE NERVOUS SYSTEM

THE object of this excursion into evolutionary and embryo-logical theory has been two-fold. First, it has been designed to shew that the pattern theory is applicable not merely to psychological, nor to physiological, phenomena, but also may have, perhaps, a general biological reference. That the reconstruction of evolution I have outlined is the correct one I would not claim, but that the pattern theory can be applied to the facts in some such way I am confident. The old biological adage, "Ontogeny is a brief recapitulation of phylogeny", seems to me to be in the language of "patterns", and not in that of preformism or of epigenesis, while the pattern theory covers the facts brought forward by both these schools. The second object has been to give a rational introduction to a discussion of the relationship between structure and function in the nervous system. This will involve the fabrication of some hypothesis as to the development of the nervous system.

When the anatomy of the central nervous system is studied, the complexities of interconnection between ganglion cells by dendrites and axones and between regions by tracts is bewildering and astounding. To account for this epigenetically various authors have attempted explanations that are mechanical (His), electrical (Strasser, Kappers, Child), or chemical (Cajal). Of these, the most interesting is that of Kappers, who has developed a theory of "neurobiotaxis", that has been slightly modified by Child.[1] The evidence on which this is based is derived from embryological observations and deduced from studies of the comparative anatomy of the nervous system. According to this theory, a stimulus creates an electrical field, spreading out from the point of origin into the surrounding lymph. A neuroblast lying in this

[1] See Child's *Origin and Development of the Nervous System* for references to Kappers' papers.

field will suffer a resulting polarization. Differences of potential are thus set up within it, which produce a physiological gradient in the cell, and this, in turn, provokes differential growth: the dendrites grow towards the stimulus and the axones away from it. Ingvar[1] has given some experimental support to this theory by determining the direction of outgrowth of nerve cells in tissue cultures with an electric current. Further description of neuro-biotaxis would carry us into technicalities inappropriate to this book. It should merely be pointed out that it is an attempt to account for the morphology of the nervous system as a response to function, and as a response that is purely mechanical, i.e. a blind and inevitable result of physico-chemical factors.

As is usual with such explanation, however, it is one thing to shew how a single neurone may grow differentially, or move in response to a stimulus, and another thing to account for the presence and selective action of stimuli that will produce a complicated network of interlacing fibres, each one of which has its correct destination and adult connections.

Bok has gone some way towards solution of this problem with his theory of stimulogenous fibrillation.[2] He made a painstaking study of the development of the paths in the brain stem of chick embryos and, from the order of appearance of the different elements and their behaviour relative to one another, deduced that they were by their activity effecting the growth of their interconnections. His theory, in brief, is that repeated passage of stimuli causes nerve fibrils to be laid down along the path of excitation. If two centres are excited at the same time, or in immediate succession, the disturbance radiates out from both and, of course, is greatest in the line between them. (Kappers had already claimed this in 1908 in the words, "Das Grundgesetz der Psychologie, ein Grundgesetz der Hirnanatomie".) Along this line nerve fibrils are laid down. This means in turn a greater flow of impulses along the line which is now a path. The neuro-fibrils not being insulated at this period, the excitations spread out into the surrounding tissue, and such other neuroblasts migrate towards it as are already excited, so that new connections are

[1] "Reaction of Cells to the Galvanic Current in Tissue Cultures", *Proc. Soc. Biol. and Med.* vol. xxxiv, 1921.
[2] "Die Entwickelung der Hirnnerven und ihrer zentralen Bahnen. Die Stimulogene Fibrillation", *Folia Neurobiologica*, 1915, vol. ix, p. 475.

built up. The process is thus cumulative, but at each stage depends on function.

To account for the final complexity, Bok falls back on the mneme theory: the stimuli are received in countless consecutive generations, gradually causing the differentiation of more and more paths. He says: "According to this hypothesis, the formation of fibrils is connected wholly with the general property of protoplasm to adapt itself to repeated stimulation: the axones and dendrites—possibly the neurofibrils contained therein—are the strongest, microscopically visible engrams". No clearer presentation of the mneme theory could be found than this, and its inadequacy is obvious on a moment's consideration. The engram is not something immaterial like an image function or pattern. It is a record written physico-chemically into the protoplasm: it is even visible! Yet this visible structure is the carrier of past experience from one generation to another in spite of the fact that it only appears comparatively late in embryological development. If it be a visible structure, where is it in the egg?[1] This is the point of fatal weakness in the mneme theory. If, however, for engram in the physical sense we read "growth pattern", Bok has provided an hypothesis of the development of the nervous system analogous to, and at points identical with, what I am now going to propose.

In unicellular organisms there might be a temporary differentiation of some strands of protoplasm for the purpose of conduction, but the variability of shape of the organism, or the variations of functions performed by such parts as may have become morphologically differentiated, preclude the development of really specialized nervous tissue. The function of conduction may be considerably improved but, failing the repetition of impulses over an identical path, the appearance of true nerves is not to be expected.

In primitive multicellular organisms, on the other hand, certain cells in the mass may conduct more impulses on account of their

---

[1] A defence might be attempted by stressing the importance of the stimuli arising from the developing nerve cells for the differentiation of others—the neurobiotaxic theory. But for some developments this is an inconceivable factor. For example, what stimulus leads to the outpouchings of the fore-brain that form the optic vesicles with their peculiar shape and peculiar effects on the skin and mesodermal tissues? No light reaches the embryonic brain. Some kind of a growth pattern must be operating.

position in the line of conduction from the part of the body most exposed to stimulation. If conduction depends on the building up of differences of potential on the two sides of a permeable membrane, this ought, on my theory, to follow as a repair reaction whenever an impulse is propagated continuously, and gradually to cause a differentiation of nervous tissue, as the repeated repair is integrated into a growth pattern.

The type of nervous system arising in this way consists of one or a few ganglion cells from which long nerve processes run to distant parts of the body. It is characteristic of the invertebrates. It should be noted that the nerve cells and processes lie in the general cell masses of the body. They can, therefore, only function in such a special chemical medium as can be maintained by the thin sheaths of the nerves. This means that a limit is placed on their specialization and that conduction remains relatively slow. In vertebrates—including mammals—this type remains in the involuntary nervous system, the reactions of which are slower than in the nerves of the voluntary system in the same species.

Another and higher type appears with segmentation. If we assume that a series of animals, each with such a nervous system containing a number of nerve cells, coalesce, then the cross connections between the ganglion cells of one segment and the other segments will produce a network within what is now the central nervous system. This reconstruction is, of course, artificial, for the complication of the nervous system of each segment develops *pari passu* with the appearance of segmentation and the elaboration of appendages (locomotory, etc.) serving the organism as an integrated whole. The hypothetical segments that first come together would have only a few nerve cells, being possessed of few differentiated structures. The point is, however, that it is the combinations of segmental systems which make possible—and indeed render inevitable—a great complication of nervous elements which is the *sine qua non* of a central nervous system.

Our next problem is the differentiation of structure within the central nervous system for local and for multisegmental responses. The chief reactions of a primitive segment will have been ingesting food and withdrawing from injury. Food in the "mouth" will always send stimuli to the same part of the nerve mass; swallowing will always employ the same channels of efferent impulses. These will gradually develop at the expense of other possible functions, until there are afferent and efferent nerves and an eating centre. On the other hand, every part of the body wall is connected with the nervous system and is liable to harm. Retraction from a noxious stimulus is something first occurring in the local protoplasm. If one part were exposed to injury more than the rest of the body surface, no differentiation of nervous tissue for this function could occur; but if one point were constantly injured, such as the end of a limb structure, then there would be an integration of the local reaction with the local stimulus as a nervous rather than protoplasmic reaction. When segments coalesce, eating reflexes take on the passage of food through a continuous gut. The oesophagus, for example, acts segmentally. Nociceptive reactions remain segmental, unless the segments coalesce in the formation of a common limb structure. Then the nociceptive reaction becomes, inevitably, a co-ordinate one. But segmental traces remain as is seen in the local signature of the flexion reflex in a spinal dog. Stimulation of the inner or of the outer side of the foot produces different reflexes, the stimulated point tending to be moved farther than the opposite side of the foot.

Repetition of identical reactions will lead to structural specialization. We can conceive, then, of structure shewing such parallellism with very simple primitive reactions that the latter would seem to be direct expression of the former. We might have, for example, a reflex mechanical structure like that of text-book diagrams, if some spot of the skin were being continually stimulated and leading to identical muscle contraction time after time, and if this muscle did not participate in any other reflex.

The artificiality of this scheme is shewn, however, if we consider a muscle in the leg of such a neurologically undeveloped creature as the frog. That muscle moves in at least four reflexes—hopping, flexion, wiping[1] and righting. The only part of the nervous structure identical in all is the path from the central nervous system to the muscle, i.e. the nerve. Here structural specialization is complete and the function of the muscle is wholly dependent on the integrity of the motor nerve. We could imagine a separate

[1] Wiping is a reflex seen even in the spinal frog to have extraordinary localization. If a drop of acid be placed on the skin of the trunk, the hind leg of that side will wipe at the spot accurately. If that leg be held, the other hind leg will reach up to perform the same task, and if it be mechanically impossible for the leg to reach the spot, attempts will still be made to do so.

localized constellation of neurones governing each of these reflexes, but were this so, localized injury in the lumbar cord would knock out only one reflex. But the only way in which one reflex is ever eliminated is by cutting off the lumbar cord from its connections with the head region that subserve some general function, like that of balance. A spinal reflex, having its whole *raison d'être* in balance, will then disappear. We are, therefore, forced to the view that the neurones providing stimuli to the efferent nerves are interconnected, or at least spatially intertwined. As they inhibit one another, some kind of interconnections must exist. Further, the regulating neurones must have a wide area of distribution. Flexion could be confined to the lumbar cord, but the other reflexes involve many segments—locomotion (integrated with sight, smell and sound stimuli), righting (depending on labyrinthine stimuli), and wiping (having all the skin of the body as its receptive field). Wide distribution does not, of course, preclude the possibility of specific structure, but variations and gradations of response do. If there are specific sets of neurones, there must be many such for each "type" reflex. The localization of wiping, for example, not to mention crossed wiping, is difficult to explain by one mechanism. Since reflexes are not always the same, there could, according to my developmental theory, be no specific structure for determining them.

Another argument is more important on account of the theoretic principles involved therein. The voluntary nervous system of vertebrates and their musculature are developed in connection with locomotion. The primitive function of withdrawal from noxa utilizes muscles developed in connection with more specialized functions and, therefore, probably utilizes the nervous control of these later structures as well. Or, more likely, each utilizes primitive segmental nerve-muscle structures subserving both functions. Under these circumstances, entirely separate neurone constellations for different reflexes is almost unthinkable, after that point in evolution is reached where the weight of the body is taken by legs. The reason for this is as follows: The leg now has two equally important functions, to support the weight of the body and to move it. Neither of these functions can exist in one leg independently of the others. If one leg be lifted, at least one other must take the weight that is left unsupported. Support and locomotion are, then, co-ordinated functions and this co-ordination is as inevitable as that one arm of a balance goes up when the other goes down. The co-ordination involves many proprioceptive stimuli from both of a pair of opposed legs. Now, if flexion and stepping developed side by side independently, and each had its own crossed co-ordination, then there would still be a good deal of overlapping, for the proprioceptives of one reaction would very nearly duplicate those for the other. This would lead to flexion activating stepping as well, unless the proprioceptive systems were quite independent. If interdependent, there would be an inter-locking of the two neurone mechanisms of the afferent side. Ex-periments shew that flexion does tend to lead over into stepping. Sherrington[1] concludes from a study of crossed extension rebound that there is a natural tendency for contraction of the flexor group of muscles in the hind leg to lead over into extension; this is stepping. (This is one of the phenomena I have cited as an ex-ample of an image function.) We must, therefore, conclude that flexion and locomotion cannot have even hypothetically separate mechanisms.

Now, the hind legs move in conjunction with the front ones, and stimuli for these movements come from the projicient centres. Balance involves proprioceptive stimuli from all four limbs, the trunk and the labyrinth. Therefore, the anatomical designs in the intact animal—even for withdrawing a hind leg from injury—operate throughout the length of the central nervous system axis from the midbrain back to the lumbar enlargement.

If flexion—taking it as an example—is not functionally separate from reactions involving the whole central nervous system axis, why does it appear in the spinal animal at all? The answer is that the withdrawal-from-injury-reaction just discussed, with its wide anatomical representation and its functional co-ordination, does disappear in the spinal animal. It is a more or less discrimi-native response. In its place appears a non-discriminative one known as the flexion reflex. But, it might be argued, why is the spinal reflex inco-ordinate and non-discriminative? According to my theory, even the highly discriminative reactions are guided by patterns. These patterns have already been formed. Patterns are immaterial, therefore no operation on the central nervous system will destroy them. For their expression a design is needed, how-ever. This design is a relationship between neurones in a state of

[1] *Proc. Roy. Soc.* B, 1908, pp. 68, 69.

excitement, having been stimulated thereto by afferent impulses. In the spinal animal the necessary afferent neurones are present; the efferent neurones and muscles are also intact. Surely, the spinal cord contains enough connector neurones to express the design specific for the discriminative response, when directed by a pattern that is indestructible. According to this reasoning, then, the spinal animal ought to be able to perform discriminative responses to tactile stimuli, which it plainly cannot do. Ought we not to assume, perhaps, that the flexion reflex is a function of a mechanical system of neurones in the lumbar cord, which produces this reflex when the cord is isolated, just as the wheels and hands of a clock will buzz wildly round when the pendular control is removed. These are crucial questions.

The first point to be borne in mind is that we are not dealing with what patterns there might be, but with the ones that really are. The patterns for discriminative flexion are composed of a series of flexions to each one of which there is added a qualifying element. This might be represented as *abc, abd, abe, abf*, etc. The qualifying element is associated with some reaction serving the animal as a whole. The behaviour of the total animal is behaviour relative to the environment, and the stimuli which call forth such integrated reflexes reach the animal through the projicient senses. It is sight, smell, or sound (together with gravitational or kinetic impressions in the labyrinth) which elicits the qualitative response. Discriminative reactions must, then, be guided by patterns of the intact animal. Conceivably, a species with only a spinal cord might in time develop patterns for discriminative response to tactile stimuli alone, but actually the mammals we study have not. The discriminative movement of a limb is essentially part of a projicient pattern.

On the other hand, in a series of discriminative movements directed to quite divers ends there may be certain elements that constantly recur. For instance, if the *ab* of the series *abc, abd, abe, abf*, etc., be flexion and crossed extension, these recur in the intact dog in the flexion reflex, in the scratch reflex, in stepping and in running. The repetition of these two elements will cause them to be conditioned together, in so far as the movements are identical in a sufficiently long series, and the combination can be adaptive by itself. In an animal that lay on its belly, crossed extension would not occur with flexion, so the extension must have originated as part of a widespread balancing reaction. The same thing is true of the crossed extension with the scratch reflex. But once an integration between the two is effected, the more automatic (i.e. the more independent of projicience) it becomes, the better it is for the animal. The sub-pattern *ab* may, therefore, have enough of a separate existence to allow of its resurrection after the projicient patterns lapse.

In so far as flexion, *qua* flexion, may be liberated in all the more complicated reactions containing it by precisely the same neurones, to that extent would there develop, according to my scheme, a specialized structure for flexion in the spinal cord. But in order that this should be, every act of flexion in a series of generations must have involved just the same constellation of neurones. If there have been variations, only such neurones will be structurally united as have been invariably and exclusively excited. In other words, it is only that small element constant to all acts of flexion that would gain specific structural representation in the cord. And the flexion observed in the spinal animal is a much larger affair than this.

I have claimed that complicated patterns may be activated by obvious stimulation of only some of their elements, images acting as the stimuli for the remaining ones. With an isolated cord an animal has all its muscles, the full equipment of motor and sensory nerves, and a considerable mass of grey matter in its cord, enough to provide an ample network of neurones for many complicated reactions. Why, then, on my theory, should not the immaterial, and therefore indestructible, complicated patterns of the intact animal be able to find expression in the spinal animal? The answer is that image functions do appear, one unit reaction may lead to others, as has occurred in the intact animal, but that these later ones are not co-ordinated. For instance, flexion in the hind limb may lead to flexion or extension in one or both fore limbs, or to stepping movements in the same or opposed hind limbs, but these are never co-ordinated. The spinal animal does not succeed in walking away from the noxious stimulus. Why not? This leads to a consideration of the relationship between "higher" and "lower" regions of the central nervous system anatomically, and the meaning of this in terms of patterns.

The first point is the nature of the connection anatomically. This is by tracts. Their origin may be accounted for as in the case of peripheral nerves. Let us suppose that there is a more or less undifferentiated matrix of conductive tissue in what is going to become the bulbo-spinal axis. A stimulus received in the caudal end reaches the oral extremity, and *vice versa*. Patterns are being built up gradually as wider and wider co-ordinations. The more integrated these patterns become, i.e. the more they govern the body as a whole, the oftener will impulses be going in a longitudinal direction, joining segment to segment, and connecting the distant structures that are thus brought into a functional unity. A result is that in an innumerable series of reactions the same pathways will be traversed in the service of diverse reactions. This is because the same muscular structure makes countless different movements. Roughly a score of muscles, for example, move the human hand, but who could place a limit to the movements it may make? There will then be a constant repetition of stimuli going from the head centres to a limited number of "centres" in the cord. If a continuance of conduction over a given path means differentiation of structure along that path, the appearance of a tract along this pathway would result inevitably.

Once tracts have appeared, a greater speed of reaction is possible, and this facilitates new co-ordinations. The latter are the more complicated patterns that lapse in the isolated cord. But the degree of loss varies with different species. It is greatest in man, a fact difficult to account for anatomically, since there is no evidence of the spinal cord in man being less specialized anatomically than in the dog, for example. The pattern theory may explain this, however.

In the head are the organs of special sense that belong peculiarly to the organism as a whole and not to segments. These are the labyrinth for balancing, the ear for hearing, the eyes for vision, and the nose for smell. They maintain equilibrium and direct movements. With the exception of the labyrinth, all deal with stimuli that originate at a distance from the body, and are hence called projicient by Sherrington. He shews how the brain has developed in connection therewith: The function of a central nervous system is co-ordination, and co-ordination is useful in adapting the organism to its environment. Therefore, most reactions of a central nervous system (particularly in higher animals) will be concerned with the outer world. Organs and nerves that bring in the most useful (and, therefore, the most used) stimuli will develop most. This is the explanation of there being more fibres in one optic nerve than in all the afferent spinal roots of one side. It follows from this that by far the greatest bulk of the impulses coming in to the cerebro-spinal axis will be at the oral end. Since structure follows function (as I would say), the oral end is the one that develops the brain.

Adaptation to the environment is what necessitates a modification of patterns. The degree of modification will vary greatly. A horse can shake off a fly by twitching its skin, a reaction that does not need the co-operation of any head organs, and does not interfere with any adaptation of the body as a whole; so that can be a purely spinal function. A dog lying on its side can scratch at a fly. No head organs are necessarily involved in the task of localizing the fly; hence the scratch reflex may be purely spinal and be accurate. On the other hand, if the dog be standing when the fly alights, to scratch may upset its balance. Recognition and correction of this involves labyrinthine functions, so that the scratch reflex has not a pattern wholly unintegrated with more discriminative ones. However, three legs will support him; so a single shift of the other hind leg may become a perfectly routine operation, and be perfectly integrated with the scratching movements, ceasing to be discriminative. Hence, there is a crossed extension with scratch as a spinal reflex. On the other hand, rising on both hind legs is a reaction prompted only by sight or smell. No spinal dog exhibits double extension in its hind legs.

Let us now compare with this the situation of a man. What reactions has he into which head-organ stimuli do not enter? There are visceral ones, of course, and these all survive a total lesion of the cord, even when they include elaborate movements of voluntary muscles, as in the coitus reflex. The movements of the upper extremity are all of the discriminative order, and they lapse when the cord is isolated. (It is difficult, of course, to get data as to these, for a total lesion of the spinal cord in man high enough to isolate all the arm centres is followed by protracted shock, and death is apt to occur before the shock may have had time to disappear.) One might, perhaps, expect the more un-discriminative reflexes of the legs to survive. In man, however, walking, or even standing, involves the constant use of the laby-rinth and eyes. Hence, he has no reflexes exhibiting a co-ordination of both legs in the purely spinal state. A part of the flexion reflex in the dog is crossed extension. This is present in man only when some connections with the higher centres persist.[1] Flexion may even spread to the other leg—a more purely segmental kind of action than any observable in the spinal dog.

One question remains to be answered: Why are image functions that appear in the spinal animal not co-ordinated? Spinal cord reflexes are essential component parts of co-ordinated responses; patterns to integrate these have been long since perfected. Why does the spinal dog not walk away from the pin that pricks his foot, why do only inco-ordinate movements suggesting walking appear? The answer comes from our laws of patterns as deduced from pyschology. The effectual stimulus for a complicated integration of patterns is the goal. On the neurological level, this means a discriminative response to an adaptive need, i.e. a response to a stimulus different from any of those which liberate the unit elements making up the complicated reaction. Walking is directed towards a smell, sight, or sound and the co-ordination of balance refers not to the welfare of any one of the legs but of the body as a whole. The effective stimuli, therefore, for co-ordinated movements of progression and of balancing are stimuli from the nose, eyes, and ear organs. This is where the close analogy between the control of images by consciousness and of spinal image functions by the operations of the encephalon appears. An image uncontrolled by consciousness is an hallucination, i.e. something not co-ordinated with the adaptation of the personality. An image function of the cord leads to a random movement not co-ordinated with the adaptation of the organism as a whole.

In this connection, I might mention some interesting correlations in human spinal cases. The cord may be severely injured, so that there is complete anaesthesia, and yet some local signature may exist, such as the eliciting of extension instead of flexion by scratching the thigh. This is recognized by Riddoch as a sign of some connection with the higher centres still persisting. Correlated with this is an inhibition of the reflex spread. Flexion is then more localized to the limb stimulated and facilitation of the bladder evacuation reflex does not occur. With this degree of injury crossed extension also appears. In other words, there is inhibition on the one hand and the more elaborate pattern on the other. This was

[1] An exception to this should be mentioned: Riddoch (*loc. cit.*) in two out of eight cases observed a slight crossed extension (contraction of the quadriceps and less often of the calf muscles) but of insufficient strength to move the limb.

shewn most prettily in a case with local signature in one leg and not in the other. Stimulation of the limb without it led to mass reactions, which did not occur on stimulation of the opposite side. My interpretation of this would be that the noxious stimulus sets up a train of image functions, uncontrolled by higher centres, but only of that primitive order belonging to human spinal patterns. On the side without local signature, the designs for these have no neural connection with higher centres and are uninhibited. On the other side, where these connections do exist, the image functions are controlled and activate the next higher series of patterns —those of the spinal quadruped. Hence crossed extension is obtained.

Before leaving the question of the functions of the isolated cord, one possible objection should be met. Why, if patterns be immaterial, should the connection between cord and brain matter be at all? The immaterial surely does not need any local habitation! But my theories are not spiritistic. The physiological patterns are relations and correlations of physical phenomena. They guide impulses in the central nervous system; they do not transport them. They are integrations of processes using physical means for their expression; they have developed from physical reactions, and they cannot have any demonstration without matter to express them. Every integral part of a physiological pattern is a representation of a physical phenomenon, the work of the pattern is merely the arrangement of these parts. If rapid conduction of an impulse from the sole of the foot to the midbrain has been an integral part of the pattern, that pattern cannot be demonstrated (although it may exist, metaphysically) without continuity in the appropriate nerve fibres. No more can a melody printed on paper or present in the mind of a pianist make music in a piano without hands on the keyboard. The music and the playing of the music are two different things.

Another point should be borne in mind. Speed of conduction is essential to most co-ordinations. When practice perfects a conducting structure, new co-ordinations are possible. These, then, have speed as an essential component. A mechanism not capable of speed is incapable of expressing the new function. An analogy with two games, one of which has been derived from the other, may make this point clearer. The original game of tennis is played in a court having a stone floor and stone walls and the walls are used to keep the ball in play. The ball is a heavy bundle of woollen rags, having little resiliency, and the racquets are small and heavy. From this game was derived that of lawn tennis when the discovery of india rubber made possible the invention of the light and highly resilient pneumatic ball. The speed and resilience of this ball eliminated the walls from the game, so that, according to the rules of lawn tennis, a ball may be out of play if it crosses the boundary line. Lawn tennis has thus become an entirely different game from its parent. If one now tried to play the game of lawn tennis with tennis balls and tennis racquets on the soft ground of a lawn tennis court, there would be no game at all, for the ball would never rise high enough from the ground to be hit by the player receiving it. An observer might say that "lawn tennis" had ceased to exist. The patterns for playing lawn tennis would still be present, but their expression would have become impossible.

In general, it is safe to state that the higher, more elaborate and complicated co-ordinations become, the more essential for their performance is speed of conduction. Intellectual operations represent the highest degree in development of such co-ordinations. A consequence of this is of fundamental importance in understanding the symptoms of generalized injuries to the brain. When these occur speed of conduction must be diminished and this accounts for a number of specific symptoms appearing with what is known as a mental tension defect. This, however, is a problem belonging to a later stage of our work.

CHAPTER XXVI

SUMMARY OF PHYSIOLOGICAL PATTERNS

A. *Anatomical Expression of Patterns in the Central Nervous System.*

(1) In the Central Nervous System not suffering from shock, impulses wander freely from neurone to neurone; their distribution is guided by patterns.

(2) The physical correlate of a specific nervous function is the excitation of a series of connector neurones in a specific *design*, which owes its specificity to the relationship in space and time of the unit excitations and not to the excitation of specific individual neurones. This anatomical design is a four-dimensional pattern which can be represented by the excitation of different neurones, or of a varying number of neurones: so long as enough neurones are excited to represent the design, it is irrelevant how many or what particular neurones are excited.

(3) The essence of an anatomical design is the contrast between the excitation of the neurones involved and the quiescence of the surrounding neurones.

(4) A design in full activity is the correlate of an image function; a design in semi-activity corresponds to a liminal image.

B. *Summary of Relationships between patterns and structure in the Nervous System.*

(1) At whatever level one begins to examine biological phenomena some patterns are already found to be in operation. Repetition of reaction, itself determined by pre-existent patterns, specializes the structure which participates in the reaction.

(2) For specialization to be complete and exclusive, identical reactions must be mediated by the structure, and the structure must not participate in other reactions.

(3) When structural specialization is complete, the reaction is so perfected as to make possible a new pattern, but the new function is then dependent on the integrity of the structure, together with

the operation of pre-existent more primitive functions. The reasons
for this are:

(*a*) Specialization means greater speed of conduction and the
latter makes possible new co-ordinations.

(*b*) A mechanical element, a rapidly conducting structure—or,
rather a property inherent in a mechanical element—has become
an integral and essential part of the reaction, and is that which
gives it its peculiar characteristic, just as the mechanical structure
of the limb affects the way in which a reflex is carried out. In
other words, patterns control the distribution of impulses, but
the speed of their distribution is a function of specialized structure.
(This is important for the correlation of mental tension defect
symptoms with general physical insults to the brain.)

(*c*) Interference with conduction that is essential to a pattern of
co-ordination, prevents expression of that pattern.

(4) Development of neurones occurs at such parts of the central
nervous system as receive impulses essential for the stimulation of predominant patterns, i.e. patterns occurring most frequently. (The frequency is determined largely by the selection
of stimuli consequent on pre-existent patterns, which produce an
orientation of organisms towards certain stimuli selectively. For
example, the development of projicient senses.)

(5) This makes possible the expression of more patterns allied
to the first ones: hence the integration of the later ones and their
subsequent reaction on the development of neurones. The growth
of parts of the central nervous system may, therefore, be cumulatively progressive and result in "centres", i.e. areas, essential to
the performance of certain functions.

(6) If complicated patterns be formed by combinations of
functions peculiar to a "higher" centre on the one hand, and a
"lower" centre on the other, such that the functions of the higher
centre continually modify the reaction carried out by the lower
(i.e. a series of patterns in which the pattern as a whole is invariably
modifying the subsidiary elements belonging to the lower centre),
then anatomical isolation of the two centres will abolish the
function of the lower centre. This will happen even although
anatomically the lower centre retains the afferent, connector and
efferent elements necessary for the co-ordination represented in
the subsidiary pattern.

(7) On the other hand, if complicated patterns be formed by

the combination of functions operating through higher and lower centres, such that, in a series of such patterns, the reactions of the lower centre remain constant, then anatomical separation of the higher and lower centres will not abolish the subsidiary pattern. (Cf. in the psychological field, the automatic use of "please" and "thank you", which becomes independent of the personality.)

(6) and (7) may be put symbolically: If A and B be two lower centre reactions, B being the second and originally mediated by a function C originating in a higher centre, then there may be two types of series. In the first series, we have $ACB, AC'B', AC''B''$, $AC'''B'''$, etc., and in the second series, $ACB, AC'B, AC''B$, $AC'''B$, etc. Elimination of C from the total integration will leave AB only in the second type, because in it B has followed after A often enough for the two reactions to have become integrated together as AB.

(8) Phenomena called "inhibition" are not explicable in terms of specific neural mechanisms, but are a corollary of pattern functions. A neural design involves not only certain neurones being active but that others should be relatively passive. The latter means an absence of liminal images and, therefore, a high threshold for activation of such a silent area, since liminal images must be built up first. This may be accomplished by the mechanical spread of powerful impulses.

(9) Higher centres do not inhibit lower ones but, normally, lower ones operate only in combination with the higher. Exceptions are:

(a) If the central nervous system distribution of a lower function is short and the higher reaction involves a long distance of conduction for impulses, there may be a brief appearance of the lower reaction before the combined one appears.

(b) If the combined reaction be not well integrated, either may be elicited by the same stimulus and the lower will tend to occur except when the combined reaction is already present as a liminal image. The latter comes from the presence of integrations still higher than those already active.

(10) Different parts of the central nervous system can work independently only when their functions do not overlap, i.e. contribute to more complicated functions having incompatible ends.

CHAPTER XXVII

CONCLUDING REMARKS

THIS chapter is essentially a postscript, for it stands apart from my general programme. A preliminary statement of the "pattern theory" has been given, and readers, who are conversant with the psychological, physiological or biological fields that I have skimmed over, will long since have arrived at a conclusion as to the value or uselessness of the proposed formulae. The layman, however, has not the same facility in judging of their utility. It is, therefore, desirable to "stake out my claims" in general terms, as can only be done in a concluding chapter. But this is not all. A few readers may ask the question: If the proposed formulae imply a general biological theory, what further, philosophical, implications may there not be? I cannot resist the temptation of answering this question, unqualified though I am to undertake speculations that involve metaphysics, physics and mathematical philosophy. So, because I distrust amateur philosophizing, I am anxious to dissociate these further ruminations from the main body of the work.

The first matter to be considered is the usefulness of a proposed vocabulary in psychology. Reference has been made in the Preface to the diversity in basic theory which psychologists display. This is due, I imagine, chiefly to the fact that different modes of approach yield data that belong to different orders and so cannot be easily correlated, while, at the same time, each group of phenomena is extensive enough to be capable of internal correlation and of building into a system of sufficient dignity to convince its exponent that it is a psychology by itself. Thus the introspectionists, dealing only with the data of consciousness, fabricated a system that compensated with an internal consistency for its failure to explain many human actions. An idealized being was envisaged, having a consciousness that controlled the body and itself with divine efficiency. But this creature could not have been a character, even in the most boring of Victorian novels. In the meantime dramatists, fable makers and aphorists were making shrewd remarks about human nature. Then came the psycho-pathologists, chiefly Freud and his followers, who focussed their attention on what consciousness failed to note, or was powerless to prevent. They assume an "unconscious" as the real thinker and doer, and account satisfactorily for what introspective psychology fails to explain; but they produce as their paradigm a creature in comparison with whom the hero of a Russian novel seems as tame as a Victorian curate. They are like the introspectionists, however, in treating the mind as if it were something as separable from the body as is the driver from his car. Both groups—in theory, if not in practice—dissociate mind and body, so that the latter seems to be used by the former as if it were an instrument or machine for the realizing of desires or purposes that arise on the mental level and are expressible in purely mental terms. This is perhaps defensible as a working method so long as we are dealing with adult human beings, but in children and the higher animals a consider-able portion of behaviour is seemingly the product of reflexes, and the lower one goes in the scale of animal life the more facile does physiological method become. In reversing the survey, it looks as if the mental evolved out of the physiological. Genetic psychology is, therefore, forced to begin at a level where physiological method and physiological vocabulary are preferable to the methods and vocabulary of the psychology that studies conscious man. The behaviourists have seized on the genetic method and seek to esta-blish psychology on a physiological basis: they treat the organism as if it were merely a body, a machine of extraordinary intricacy, a congerie of interrelated functions evoked by external and internal stimuli, but not regulated by any higher agency such as the layman would call the mind. The "psychology" of the behaviourists comprises only a study of the externally directed or expressed functions of the organism, but it is surprising to see how much of the adaptation of a normal average man to his environment can be expressed adequately in behaviouristic terms and his reactions explained as reflexes, instincts and habitual responses. This is equivalent to saying that the presence or absence of conscious-ness is irrelevant to an understanding of a large part of human behaviour and it may, therefore, be eliminated on the principle of parsimony. Were the whole of human behaviour explicable along these lines, the behaviourists' system would be a more defensible one than it is. Nevertheless, they have contributed much to psychology.

Criticisms similar to these could be made of other "systems" of psychology: in these, as in the cases I have considered, a particular method reveals an enormous body of phenomena, out of which a hypothetical man is built who seems to his creator to be a real man, because he has so many interrelated characteristics. In every case, however, the hypothetical creature falls short of being a true man: in other words, each system of psychology is inadequate. An adequate system should harmonize the findings of the various schools. But this, so far, no one has succeeded in doing, because the nomenclature of each school is designed only for a description of the phenomena it has elected to study. The faculty psychologists have no vocabulary in which to describe the reactions of a suckling child without making quite unjustifiable assumptions, and quite similarly the psycho-analysts to fit these responses into their system assume the existence at birth of perceptions and wishes that are inconceivable without prior experience. In describing this early stage of human life, however, the behaviourists can use the terminology involving no such assumptions. But how can a behaviourist account for the mental processes that elaborate a theory or compose a poem? So long as the data collected by different methods are formulated in terms peculiar to the methods in question, it will be impossible to synthesize all the data except in an intuitive fashion.

The pattern nomenclature may, however, offer a way out of this *impasse*. A pattern, *qua* pattern, carries with it no implications as to whether its expression will be in bodily activity, or in unconscious, or in conscious mental processes. It is, therefore, possible to translate into terms of patterns the findings of all psychological investigations, no matter what may be the methods employed in making the observations. In this translation, there is one fundamental assumption, or implication, but it is one that forces correlation and prohibits dissociation of data. This is the principle of integration. Every pattern is formed by the integration of simpler elements, and every pattern may itself become a unit in a still higher integration. "Physiological" patterns have to do with the integration of reflexes. These complexes can be associated in more and more complicated patterns, until gradually a complication is reached, which makes their classification as "mental" more expedient than as simply physiological. Yet the transition—when put into terms of patterns—is gradual, and, indeed, with this nomenclature sufficiently elaborated and familiar, it would be possible to drop the classifications physiology and psychology altogether: we should cease to speculate as to whether the mind controlled the body or the body manufactured the mind and should think only of a unitary complex of "body-mind" functions. A corollary of this is important. Every pattern being an integration of parts, the parts are implicit in the whole. Consequently, any mental event, when put in terms of patterns, includes bodily processes in the background. For instance, the most abstract idea which affects the consciousness of a philosopher may be accounted for as an integration of simpler ideas, these in turn are a correlation of perceptions, the perceptions arise as a correlation of reflexes, and at this point it is not unprofitable to think in terms of anatomical designs. Ultimately, then, analysis of the complicated ideational pattern leads to physiological elements and implies physiological activity. In this statement, there is, of course, nothing new: such a formula is the stock-in-trade of every behaviourist or materialist. But their physiology is a mechanistic one, in which functions are merely physico-chemical processes. The physiology, in my formula, is not a sum of physico-chemical processes, but an integration thereof. That is to say, it has to do with properties which appear only as a relationship of the individual processes. These processes must, however, be there before the relationship can come to expression. Dots compose the picture in a half-tone reproduction. The picture cannot be predicted from the sum of the sizes and densities of the individual dots, but is a function of their arrangement; on the other hand, without the dots there could be no half-tone picture. Metaphorically, we might say that the constitution of the individual dots is physics and chemistry; the arrangement of the dots is physiology; and the use to which the picture is put is psychology. Art cannot exist without pictures, and pictures imply the existence of material elements. Similarly, a psychological datum implies a physiological process, and that, in turn, implies physico-chemical events. According to the pattern hypothesis, however, no matter how novel the products of integration may be, there is in principle just the same thing happening when physico-chemical processes are integrated to form reflexes, when reflexes combine to make perceptions, when perceptions form ideas or ideas unite in a philosophy. And in each case the new pattern is dependent on, and implies the integrity of, a sufficient number of the subsidiary elements to represent the given relationship.

This brings us naturally to the correlation of psychopathology with psychology and physiology. Every integration, no matter how complicated, controls its subsidiary parts—so long as the integration is maintained. Within the field of psychology, there are two corollaries to this proposition which have a broad significance. The first is that, when a unitary integration suffers *dis*-integration, its component parts may appear as such and its original composition may be thus revealed. Mental disease, which is disintegration, may thus throw light on the structure of the normal mind. The second is a specific example of the first. In normal mental life, consciousness and personality are so well integrated, that a subject can usually account for his behaviour in terms of mental processes of which he is aware and has no knowledge of mental activities in addition to his conscious ones. If, however, his consciousness and personality are weakened, his actions may be determined by impulses that are not voluntary, and thoughts appear that are foreign to healthy experience. Such symptoms are held by psychopathologists to be of unconscious origin.

The concept of the unconscious owes its origin naturally enough to mental disease because, when the higher integrations exercise their normal control, exhibitions of unconscious patterns are rare, and, consequently, neglected. It might be said, indeed, that if the personality-consciousness patterns were integrated to a theoretic perfection there would be no unconscious at all: the subsidiary patterns would cease to have any expression separate from their contributions to the larger whole. As a matter of fact, however, even the most normal man experiences the effects of unconscious mental processes, as for instance in emotion, and exhibits behaviour that may be identically explained. Once the unconscious has been assumed, it provides the simplest and most adequate explanation for idiosyncratic meanings, behaviour and emotions in normal man, and has, therefore, been adopted by many academic, unprejudiced psychologists. The pattern nomenclature will serve well to ally such processes with the great mass of reactions, beginning at the physiological level, which underlie all conscious phenomena, like perceptions. This makes the "unconscious" of the psychopathologists only a part of the total mental events of which consciousness is unaware, a grouping helpful from a broad theoretic point of view but harmful if it obscures the notion of the symptom-producing unconscious having its peculiar origin and habit.

This brings us to the consideration of two different meanings given uncritically to the term "unconscious" by most psychopathologists.[1] The first is that of mental processes of which the subject is unaware, active at the time and out of harmony with the programme on which consciousness is engaged. (The last characteristic reaches its acme in "dissociation".) In the pattern nomenclature, this would be expressed by saying that the unconscious was composed of activated mental patterns not integrated with consciousness, but of the same level in the hierarchy of patterns as those which are normally integrated together to form consciousness. They belong to the same order of pattern complexity as do conscious percepts or thoughts, but are not accessible to introspection.

The other type is represented by such a mental element as the Oedipus complex. This, as I have argued in my book on Emotion, cannot be viewed as something that appears in any complete form at any period of an individual's conscious life. There is no evidence to shew that any individual, man or boy, at any time desires to have sexual intercourse with his mother and kill his father—provided each of these terms is given its literal and complete meaning. The evidence is, rather, that scattered, incomplete impulses in these directions appear in the words and deeds of childhood, and that much normal and abnormal adult behaviour and thinking can be explained satisfactorily only if we assume such a "complex" to be motivating the personality without conscious awareness thereof. But even this statement must be further qualified. The evidence does not indicate that in the adult the objects of love and hate are the real parents. The mental phenomena which are adequately explained on the basis of the "Oedipus complex" may concern the real parents, it is true; but they may be dead and always there is an expression of the tendencies towards "Mother" or "Father" people. The unconscious object comes to be an imaginary creation, an *imago*, as it is called, and the attitude unconsciously entertained towards the imago tends to be expressed

[1] An exception is Morton Prince, who discriminates between the two types as "co-conscious" and "unconscious".

in the presence (actual or imagined) of someone reminiscent of the imago. Again, these attitudes of affection and hostility contain vastly more than crude sexual and murderous lust: the difference is all that can exist between a simple instinct and an elaborate interest. Indeed, the Oedipus complex is an integration of unconscious interests. When it has been subjected to close scrutiny the evidence fails to reveal a specific incest-parricide wish, and the latter has to be recognized as a shorthand label.

Because we can label our conscious interests with specific titles we are prone to forget how fluid and indefinite they are, and to what an extent they are discovered by inference from our motives and actions. They express tendencies as much as they collate specific reactions. If this be true of conscious interests, it is still more proper to speak of complexes, having such varying expression as the Oedipus one, as mere tendencies. And the unconscious, which is composed of mere tendencies, is a difficult thing to formulate in terms of any current psychology. Freud and his followers have attempted to compose it out of elements used by introspective psychology, and have fabricated a system of wishes and fantasies which cannot satisfy a rigorous critic. Prejudiced opponents can demolish the system and then comfortably neglect the evidence. The behaviourist, doubtful as to the existence of "thoughts", feels himself secure in banning from this psychology something which never has existed as specific reaction, and for proof of which not even introspective detection is claimed. Introspective psychology itself would prefer to leave to metaphysics the question as to whether a tendency can "exist" or not. The hypothesis of the latent unconscious that harbours only potential thoughts and behaviour is something that psychologists cannot weld to any framework so far in use.

But, at this point, the pattern nomenclature may come to the rescue. A pattern is a guiding agency just as is a tendency. As such, the nature of its "existence" can be left to metaphysicians to discuss, while the psychologists can use the term as fruitfully as he can "tendency". Moreover, the problem of the formation of unconscious patterns offers no theoretic difficulty. The general description of the formation and growth of interests as given in Chapter VII is as applicable to unconscious thinking as it is to voluntary habit formation: for the formation of a pattern, it is irrelevant whether the image-functions or sub-patterns that are integrated together be conscious thoughts, represent physiological reactions, or be unconscious mental processes.

We may, indeed, go further than this. These psychological elements and strata occur in one individual, yet the evidence is strong for the existence of group reactions that cannot be dismissed as the mere algebraic sum of the reactions of the individuals in a group. There is, however, a great reluctance on the part of both psychologists and anthropologists to admit the existence of a "group mind", an opposition based apparently on the assumption of consciousness being synonymous with mind. Since the bulk of mental material with which anyone deals is found in his own mind, which he knows only through consciousness, this is a natural assumption—and prejudice. An adoption of the pattern hypothesis, however, would both abolish the prejudice and explain how there could be group reactions. Patterns, being correlations of functions and being immaterial, have no corporeal residence—if I may be allowed to speak metaphysically. Whenever any two or more reactions are repeated in relation to one another with sufficient frequency to cause their integration, a pattern is formed. If animals or men act in concert, patterns for a joint activity are formed. These patterns constitute the so-called group mind. The patterns are not individual, hence justification for the adjective group; they are mental and not physiological and are specific for the group, hence the justification for "mind". But if "mind" is going to imply consciousness the term is bad. "Group" pattern covers the phenomena and carries no unwarranted implications.[1]

We thus see that the pattern nomenclature makes possible the correlation into one system of all data with which psychology has to deal, from the reflex level up to the highest flights of human intelligence. This may be interesting enough theoretically, but what is its utility? The answer to this question is naturally to be discovered in the future, and, in the meantime, I can only point out how the practical value of the pattern theory may arise. In the first place, if others beside myself can make use of this system, it may be found easier to understand the interrelations of body and mind in these terms, and anything which facilitates understanding is surely practical, even if it merely makes exposition easier.

[1] There is, of course, nothing original in this statement, for it is just the notion —and terminology—of many anthropologists.

Secondly, however, there may be ground for hope that the method of abstraction of functions, which is involved in the pattern theory, may have the same kind of fruitfulness in a solution of problems in the biological field, as mathematics have had in the physical world. If, as I assume, living forms are organized as a correlation of vital functions rather than as a correlation of physico-chemical processes, then the laws of functional correlation can be transferred from one biological domain to another, just as mathematicians will carry over their laws of number and dimension from one medium to another, assuming that relationships holding in one sphere must also apply in another. It is, however, more than an assumption on their part. In so far as the generalization, or law, is concerned solely with the properties which are abstracted and correctly correlated, the same properties are bound logically to exhibit the same behaviour in another situation, provided they can be truly abstracted in the second instance as well. The last is the crucial proviso. If the reproduction of past experience that appears in embryological development, for instance, is, fundamentally, a different process from the reproduction of past experience of which I may be consciously aware, then psychological laws cannot be carried over into embryology. That they are fundamentally the same, I fully believe.

But belief is not scientific, no matter how prevalent it may be among scientists, including materialists. Science makes hypotheses and tests them by appeal to facts. Before this can be well begun, the mutual reactions of mind and body should be more fully expressed in terms of patterns. In this book space has permitted only a sketchy outline of my programme. In an ensuing volume, I hope to demonstrate the structure of mental life as an integration of simpler physiological patterns, and trace the development of this integration from stage to stage, beginning with the spinal reflexes and going on to the emergence of consciousness. I hope that, when this has been accomplished, the unity of mental and bodily processes will appear more as a theory and less as a creed.

These concluding remarks have so far concerned only the psychological and physiological aspects of the pattern hypothesis; there remain to be considered its wider applications, the first of which is to general biological theory. I have sketched an evolutionary theory which accounts for an evolved bodily structure as a product of function: function causes a loss of the material which carries out that function; the loss is more than made good by over-repair which results in time in specialized tissue; a repetition in the production of specialized tissue leads, in turn, to the establishment of a growth pattern for the structure, so that, eventually, the structure may appear in anticipation of its function. Mention has been made of the extension of these formative processes through innumerable generations, and we must now consider a corollary to this. A pattern which is integrated from the reactions of a number of individuals in a group is a group, and not an individual, pattern: in this instance the growth patterns belong to the species and not to members of it. This enables us to understand why sex cells are so independent of the body that houses them. Germ cells, whose function it is to divide and thus give rise to new individuals, belong to the species and are modifiable only as the species is modifiable. Hence the ovaries of a black rabbit when transplanted into a white doe will still produce black offspring; the colour is a function of the strain and not of the individual. Once it is realized that growth patterns are specific, and not individual, and that their medium of expression is the germ cells, then the futility of trying to prove the Lamarckian theory by experiments on higher animals or plants becomes apparent. Before heredity can be changed the reactions of the species must be altered and, until this is accomplished, no inheritance of a modification can be expected.

On the other hand, it must be borne in mind that repair is an individual function and that, therefore, growth, which is repair or improvement of individual structure, is individual. There is ontogeny which is the function of germ and embryonic cells, and there is individual structural adaptation. According to my hypothesis, the former evolves from the latter. Perfect integration implies rigidity of reaction, and an end to modification of the patterns involved. Since evolution has not ceased, we should not expect the growth patterns of the species to be the only factors in the development of the individual, and this the influence of function on development shews. The lower the form of life, the less is the ontogenetic pattern exclusive in its determination of adult form, and the larger is the rôle played by individual growth patterns. Hence, in highly specialized organisms, repair is confined to small parts of structures. For instance, a cut in a human finger may be so well repaired that the original skin architecture will be wholly reproduced. But if a terminal joint is lost, it will never be replaced. In mammals, whole structures are produced only as a part of the building of the total body. In crustaceans, however, and even in some amphibia, whole limbs may be reproduced after accidental or experimental loss, and, in flat-worms, the animal may be cut in two and two new creatures result, a new head and a new tail-piece appearing by regeneration. The conditions under which regeneration of parts will or will not appear is a fascinating field of study. I suspect that these conditions can be put into terms of the simplicity or complexity of the function of the reproduced part and of the closeness or looseness of the integration of its function with those of the organism as a whole. In this connection, we may recall the necessity for a retained nerve supply to the regenerating part, if the new structure is to have a specialized form. (Thus, the taste buds in the skin of a catfish regenerate only if the nerve supply is intact, and in the crayfish an eye will be replaced by an undifferentiated tentacle unless the nerve is left.) Nervous supply is morphological evidence of the function of the part being integrated with the functions of the organism as a whole.

The idea of treating a species as if it were a unit, is, of course, not new. Its latest exponent is von Uexküll,[1] who gravely proposes to call the species an organism. Since we are so accustomed to think of an organism as composed of parts in physical continuity, this term is probably unfortunate. The idea is fruitful, however. In fact one of its fruits is Darwin's *Origin of Species*. In his notebook of 1837 we find these words:[2]

"It is a wonderful fact, horse, elephant, and mastodon, dying out about same time in such different quarters.

"Will Mr Lyell say that some [same ?] circumstance killed it over a tract from Spain to South America?—(Never.)

"They die, without they change, like golden pippins; it is a *generation of species* like generation *of individuals*.

"Why does individual die? To perpetuate certain peculiarities (therefore adaptation), and obliterate accidental varieties, and to accommodate itself to change (for, of course, change, even in varieties, is accommodation). Now this argument applies to species.

"If individual cannot propagate he has no issue—so with species.

---

[1] J. von Uexküll, *Theoretical Biology*, London, Kegan Paul, 1926.
[2] *Life and Letters of Charles Darwin*, edited by Francis Darwin, 3rd edition, vol. II, p. 7.

"If *species* generate other *species*, their race is not utterly cut off:—like golden pippins, if produced by seed, go on—otherwise all die.

"The fossil horse generated, in South Africa, zebra—and continued—perished in America.

"All animals of same species are bound together just like buds of plants, which die at one time, though produced either sooner or later. Prove animals like plants—trace gradation between associated and non-associated animals—and the story will be complete."

When Darwin called the species an individual and treated it as such, he probably regarded the procedure as argument by analogy. In the light of the pattern hypothesis this may be rational method. If an analogy be sound it must rest on an identity in the laws of the patterns which produced the analogous phenomena. The laws which hold for one must, therefore, produce effects in the other; but in order to use the method safely it is necessary to abstract the pertinent qualities.

The true analogy in the psychological field to the species as a unit is, however, personality. This is an integration of patterns (interests) which gives a peculiar individual trend to the behaviour of the organism. Reactions pertinent to this trend are facilitated or inhibited as the case may be. Reactions irrelevant to the personality are unaffected by the general integration. At the same time, personality can change as the result of the cumulative influence of some sub-pattern (interest) which is augmented in its relative importance by constant stimulation. The modified personality has then new affinities and new apathies. These processes are all detectable in the species, if we look on the functions and forms of the individual members as the reactions whose integration constitutes the species. A variation not incompatible with the *motif* of the species can occur, but it is as irrelevant to modification of the species as is the occurrence of an isolated response to a chance stimulus in the case of personality. The latter is changed only when interests are elevated or depressed. The reactions which are peculiar to the species are those which produce the individuals thereof and they consist in the development of the germ cells. Peculiarities of development may be integrated together, as depicted in the Mendelian formulae, which correspond to the interests that affect personality. Just as a new combination of interests (sublimations) may affect personality, so a new combination of morphological variations will produce a new type. The development of the germ cells depends (in all higher animals and plants) on the mutual stimulation of the male and female elements, and it is through sex that the selection or rejection of new morphological types is effected.

Within the germ cells, again, the essential elements seem to be the chromosomes. Fertile hybrids (in wheat for instance) can be produced by crossing species having the same number of chromosomes. If a 14-chromosome species be crossed with another 14, the resulting hybrid will be fertile. If, on the other hand, a 14 form be bred with one having 21 chromosomes, the 14–21 hybrid cannot fertilize itself, but may be prolifically crossed again with a 14 or a 21 species. The 14–21 individual is artificial, like the assumption by a man of a new name which does not belong to his personality, and hence has no automatic response attached to it: it will not recur spontaneously. It is a utilization of a substitute for which no pattern is formed. On the other hand, the fertility of the cross between the 14–21 hybrid and, for example, the 14-chromosome individual, reproducing the 14 type but with traces of the 21 characteristics, is like a personality slightly modified by the addition of a new reaction. It is like a new pattern formed by the utilization of a substitute which causes a change in the reaction.

The spontaneous appearance of a new characteristic is the analogue in a psychological sphere of new reactions as a result of combinations of patterns. Whether the new pattern persists or not depends on its integration with the personality. In the science of genetics, the new patterns are called fluctuations, if temporary, or mutations, if they persist. Geneticists cannot distinguish between the two without breeding for a number of generations. It is possible that the pattern theory might point the way to a solution of this puzzle. More intelligent animals, like anthropoid apes and man, indulge the combining tendency as a kind of pastime: playful combinations would be fluctuations that fade away in a few generations. Combinations that persist do so in virtue of their integration with the personality, this, in turn, means that they repeatedly make possible the indulgence of an appetite or that they satisfy some dominant interest. The indulgence of appetites is, biologically, a condition of survival and, according to Darwin's view, spontaneous variations persist when they favour survival. *If* a fluctuation favours the vital activities of the individuals shewing it, and *if* there be a struggle for survival, then the fluctuation would tend to be integrated with the species pattern. But how often are these conditions satisfied in breeding experiments? To establish an environment in which the individuals could survive only in virtue of the fluctuation would be difficult indeed, although perhaps not always impossible. The other condition of integration with the personality of a combined pattern is that it satisfies some important interest. Now, interests are relatively independent of the immediate situation, so that integration may take place without repeated environmental influence. This, for the fluctuating animal or plant, would mean that the fluctuation represents an opportunity for exercise of a function that *historically* is important for the species. The need that is satisfied by the fluctuation is not one arising from immediate environmental stress, but is one that has been important for the species in its total history. If such a fluctuation arose it would be integrated spontaneously and be a mutation.

To many it may seem a very far cry from intelligent human reactions to the insensate modification in the colour of peas, let us say. But when these processes are put in terms of purpose, the analogy may appear closer. In each case, we are dealing with improved adaptability gained by a variability of response; and, in each case, the adaptation is for the aggrandisement of a complicated system so highly integrated that it can be treated only as an abstraction. Personality is an integration of behaviour patterns that has achieved an independence of any one of its constituent reactions. A species is an integration of anatomical and physiological patterns that has achieved an independence of any one of its constituent individuals. A personality that ceases to change is at the mercy of the changes in the environment—the tragedy of old age. A species that ceases to vary is at the mercy of the environment—like the dinosaurs specialized for the oecological setting of a temperate climate. Wherever we turn we see exclusive specialization associated with vulnerability. This is nowhere better exemplified than in the cells of our own bodies. If the skin be cut, the cells next to the dead ones will lose their specialized form, regress to a primitive type, reproduce as such in the repair reaction and then re-specialize. The skin is a relatively undifferentiated tissue as compared with the nerve cells in the brain. Once the latter have achieved their adult form, they can never reproduce themselves, and so the total number of our brain cells diminishes day by day as we grow older. Perfect specialization, perfect integration, means adaptability only towards the environment to meet which the specialization was developed.

The objection may be raised at this point that these formulations are inapplicable to man himself. In the first place, his intelligence produces new combinations that are adaptive in survival and do satisfy dominant interests and yet they are not inherited, at least not with unequivocal clearness and frequency. In the second place, man is grotesquely specialized but he survives.

The first objection is based on the conception of the human species being composed of individuals. But, biologically, man is a herd animal and, in consequence, his intellectual originalities have social rather than individual significance. And society does perpetuate the adaptively useful combination from one generation to the next by education and imitation, which are the social means of reproduction. When a peculiar mode of adaptation becomes thoroughly identified with the group, a national or racial characteristic appears and this may be transmitted by individual heredity.

The second objection may be similarly met. It is true that individual men are highly specialized but they are units in the total social organization. So long as they remain in the civilization that they fit, their specialization has a positive survival value and their society is the more adaptive the more different specializations it harbours. In fact, the adaptability of groups depends on their possession of specialized individuals. If a society becomes too homogeneous it dies. Thus, the city state of ancient Greece lost in adaptability as it gained in intellectual and artistic glory: so it died. These principles have a profound sociological significance which is apt to be lost sight of. Specialization means sterility, so the "upper" classes are bound to be less fecund than the lower ones: not only do they tend to have a lower birth rate, but they are killed off by wars and die in hazardous enterprises which it is their function to perform. If the group is to be viewed as an organism, the upper classes are the head and the lower the body, so more stupid people function as the generative organs. "And the eye cannot say to the hand, I have no need of thee: or again the head to the feet, I have no need of you." Ardent reformers would have us dispense with the feeble-minded, not merely with the idiots and imbeciles who are plainly pathological, but also with those who do not attain "mental age" of more than nine or ten years.

Yet the stupid peasant woman is the mother of the race and always will be. Eliminate her and an over-specialized, moribund race will result. The folly of modern society lies not in allowing stupid people to breed, but in putting into their hands responsibilities for which they are unfit. To follow the bodily parallel, again, this is like demanding manual dexterity from the feet, organs that ought to bear the weight of the body and carry the hands about.

In the evolutionary scheme, which I have proposed, I began with undifferentiated protoplasm. That is to say, I assumed a pre-existent life. If speculation is to be permitted to its logical extremity, the relationship of the organism to the inorganic world should be included in the survey. Before a bit of matter can be spoken of as alive, it has to exhibit certain properties which focus themselves on the capacity to maintain the organism essentially unchanged in a changing environment. This is accomplished by the processes of digestion, excretion, motility, conduction, repair and reproduction. It has frequently been pointed out that these processes do not occur solely in the organic world but are all of them represented in inorganic matter as well. This has heartened the materialists who hold that life is a summation of physico-chemical processes. Were this so, a primitive kind of life might be synthesized in a laboratory. But this view neglects the great principle of integration. It is not enough to have all these physico-chemical processes present and in their correct proportions. The processes must be integrated together to form a unit that controls the activity of each component. In all true integrations a new property appears—the principle of creative synthesis or emergent evolution—and this property is something not derivable from those of the constituent elements. Indeed, it is only in quite simple chemical combinations that the new properties can be predicted.

According to our laws of patterns, simpler and more primitive reactions are more slowly integrated than the higher ones. One would, therefore, expect that the difference of speed in formation between psychological and physiological patterns would be parallelled by a similar difference between those for specialization of living forms and the establishment of life itself. The last involves time intervals of the order with which geologists and astronomers deal. It is unlikely then that any man, or generations of men, could observe them originating. Furthermore, we should expect such a complex constellation of properties as appears in undifferentiated protoplasm to come into being gradually, two properties being first combined, then three and so on. Were this so, a pre-vital compound would not be detectable as such, but would seem to be merely an odd chemical substance. (Ferments, for example, might be looked on as specific chemical activities united with the property of rapid reproduction. Still higher in the scale we might have filtrable viruses that we regard as alive from analogy with bacteria but are really less evolved than true living matter because they have not discrete organismic form and, therefore, lack motility and conductivity. These are, perhaps, quite idle speculations but it seems possible that immunology might receive an impetus from this kind of approach.) If pre-vital compounds exist, life, and new forms of life, may be in process of creation about us and yet remain hidden from the eyes of our keenest scientists.

It will be observed that in these conjectures about the origin of life I have assumed that protoplasm comes into being as a result of the integration of physico-chemical processes which I have treated as elements capable of integration in the same way as are biological units. This assumption carries us into the sphere of metaphysical speculation, because it gives a universal dominion to patterns. In deducing the laws of formation of patterns from mental phenomena, I have traced their origin to a combination of imaginal processes or of sub-patterns that were similarly formed. In claiming that physiological and biological regulation is traceable to similar immaterial agencies, I have pointed to the inclusion of the past in the present, which is the essential of an imaginal process. This may or may not be sound argument, but at least there is some evidence that is pertinent thereto. But where in the organic world can we look for proof of past experience affecting the present reaction, except in the cases where the past reactions have left a material change that persists? Physicists might, perhaps, be able to furnish examples of inorganic "images", but certainly I am ignorant of them. Yet I am moved to assume the operation of inorganic patterns for two reasons. The first is that it rounds out the pattern theory with a comforting universality, this being an act of faith and, therefore, scientifically disreputable. The second is modern physical theory, which I possibly misunderstand.[1]

Physicists of the present day are engaged in dissecting the atom

---

[1] Being ignorant of mathematics I have had to glean what I can about modern physics from popular books. My authorities have been: Alfred Einstein,

and studying the functions of its elements. They have arrived at the conception of an atom being a solar system in miniature. A nucleus of helium and (or) hydrogen acts as a sun around which particles known as electrons revolve like planets. The properties of the different chemical elements are derivable from the constitution of the nuclei and X-rays, light, electricity and radio-activity result from disturbances in the electrons, changing from orbit to orbit or flying off into space, or from discharges of particles from the nuclei. This reconstruction has been arrived at from experiment and mathematical reasoning: it rationalizes a large number of facts and has made possible the prediction of many discoveries. But no one, of course, has seen or could see these structures; their existence is a matter of inference and their utility is measured by the necessity that a scientist may have for a system that he can visualize in imagination, or of which he can draw a diagram. Essentially, however, the nuclei and electrons are incorporations of mathematical abstractions. They express relationships in time and space, or, more properly, in space-time. Therefore, they are merely one way of expressing patterns, the patterns which govern the behaviour of the materials and processes studied. Aether, once so respectable, has been discarded, yet it has been stated that the same principles could all be put into terms of strains in a hypothetical aether, and the notion of particulate nuclei and electrons be abandoned, or rather that they would then become the strains in the aether. (In fact, during the past year physicists have been engaged, I am told, in exploiting this latter hypothesis.)

This shews that the guiding principles are mathematical abstractions and that the solar system atom is just a model to facilitate thinking about processes that are really mathematical. Furthermore, it would appear that *any* model, attempting to embody these processes in forms accessible to sensory experience, would be inaccurate, because the processes are inconceivable in terms of common sense. The shortest distance between two points may, for instance, be a curve. Space is affected by time and time by space: neither can be considered alone but only as entering into a four-dimensional "space-time". An electron may be one instant in one orbit and the next instant in another, without having "moved"

Relativity, the Special and the General Theory, London, Methuen, 6th edition, 1921; Bertrand Russell, *The A.B.C. of Atoms*, London, Kegan Paul, 1923; C. D. Broad, *Scientific Thought*, London, Kegan Paul, 1923; A. N. Whitehead, *Science and the Modern World*, Cambridge University Press, 1926.

through the intervening space. "Mass is now absorbed into energy, and the mass of a body is not by any means always constant" (Russell). "If we wish to speak of the continuous matter present *at* any particular point of space and time, we must use the term *density*. Density multiplied by volume in space gives us *mass* or, what appears to be the same thing, *energy*. But from our space-time point of view, a far more important thing is density multiplied by a four-dimensional volume of space and time; this is *action*. The multiplication by three dimensions gives mass or energy; and the fourth multiplication gives mass or energy multiplied by time. Action is thus mass multiplied by time, or energy multiplied by time, and is more fundamental than either."[1] These fundamental units are responsible for the behaviour of atoms and the behaviour of atoms makes matter. Matter that we can handle is, then, made up of processes, i.e. patterns. It is as if one said that going-up-stairs made stairs: this, of course, is not true because lumber and carpenters, as well as plans for going upstairs, are needed at this vastly higher level of inorganic patterns; but what the physicist does say, apparently, is that when matter is analysed into its ultimate units these turn out to be processes, to be immaterial.

As we have seen so frequently, an essential feature of any integration is the appearance of new properties, and these properties are derived from the way the integrated elements are combined, rather than from the elements themselves. Organic chemistry is full of examples of this. For instance, acetylene, used as an illuminating gas, is formed of equal numbers of atoms of carbon and hydrogen, but so is the aromatic liquid benzene. In the latter case, a greater number of atoms are combined in the molecule and, according to the spatial representation of the pattern, the atoms are grouped in a ring. Two compounds may be one harmless and the other poisonous, although they seem to be the same when analysed quantitatively, a slight alteration in the grouping of the atoms being held to account for the difference in behaviour of the compounds. Studies of atomic structure reveal analogous changes of function with different arrangements of the electrons. For instance, the passage of an electron from one orbit to another will alter the amount of energy in a system. If it loses energy, it will also lose mass. Uranium by giving off radiations turns into lead and so do thorium and radium itself. An interesting example

---

[1] Eddington, quoted by Russell, *loc. cit.* pp. 164–5.

of changed properties occurs in the helium nucleus. This, on many grounds, is assumed to be made up of four hydrogen nuclei and two electrons compactly grouped together. In thus uniting, the system has lost ten million times the energy involved in combustion! The stability of the helium nucleus is so great that it has been suggested that it might be an ultimate unit of matter and not composed of hydrogen nuclei and electrons at all, which shews how thoroughly unitary and indivisible a firm integration may become. This helium nucleus gives us another example of how new properties may arise with new integrations. Its constitution is, of course, expressed accurately only in mathematical formulae; and so far no satisfactory spatial representation of the pattern has been forthcoming. But, if it be made up of particles, they must have some arrangement, and the best that has been suggested is as follows: "Imagine a somewhat primitive wheel, with four spokes, and an axle that sticks out some distance to either side. Place the two electrons at the ends of the axle, and the four hydrogen nuclei at the ends of the spokes, and imagine the wheel going round with suitable velocity. (The wheel and spokes and axle are of course imaginary, and are only intended to illustrate the relative positions of the nuclei and electrons.) This gives a configuration which has a certain degree of stability, and a flattish shape which is indicated by a certain amount of experimental evidence. It seems, however, that the degree of stability in this model is less than that required to account for the fact that no known process will disintegrate a helium nucleus. There is also a difficulty as regards the size of the helium nucleus. Taking our model and applying the quantum theory to the revolutions of the hydrogen nuclei, we can determine the radius of the circle in which they move as we determined the minimum orbit in the hydrogen atom. The result is that the size of the radius should be about five million-millionths of a centimetre. This is about seventeen times too large, according to Rutherford's experimental evidence. *It is possible, nevertheless, that our model may be right, because the forces between electrons and hydrogen nuclei may obey different laws, at such very tiny distances, from those which they obey at ordinary distances.*"[1] In other words, in this stable integration there may even be new laws operating!

Examples such as these could be repeated almost indefinitely, but enough have been given, I hope, to justify the statement that

[1] Bertrand Russell, *loc. cit.* pp. 143–4. My italics.

modern physicists analyse matter down to agencies which are immaterial in their nature and that these agencies are constituted of
integrated relationships, their properties varying with the changes
of relationships. At the psychological level, we have seen that
behaviour, whether it be objectively observed or be detected as
introspective thoughts, is determined by patterns which, broadly
speaking, exhibit the same fundamental characteristics. The un-
sophisticated find it difficult to conceive of thoughts having anything material about them, and were it not for the fact of thinking
being disturbed when the brain is injured, we should probably
have no hesitancy in believing that consciousness is independent
of matter and can apprehend the immaterial directly. On the
other hand, the highly sophisticated physicist finds it impossible
to account for a matter except as a confluence of immaterial entities.
This surely leaves the way open for a metaphysic based on functions that create and then manipulate matter, and we can conceive
of an infinite series of patterns. The most primitive ones produce
the properties which affect our senses as matter; matter is composed of such excessively stable integrations, the chemical elements,
that its origin from anything else has been unsuspected until very
recently; but when the elements combine, their products are new
properties that express a pattern and not its unit components.
These patterns are what chemists deal with, and they too are so
stable that their formation cannot be observed in the span of time
available to man for study. The next step is the integration of
these chemical patterns into life, and at this point the integrations
become sufficiently complex to be unstable and modifiable during
periods of geological computation; this gives us organic evolution
which we can observe. Once life is established, the range of possible
relationships is enormously increased: organisms react not only
with inorganic matter but amongst themselves. The reactions of
even a simple organism are, therefore, extraordinarily complicated,
and when they are integrated together a system having some self-
determination is born. This self-determination is, fundamentally,
the material with which psychology works, although biological
and physiological methods are more expedient so long as in-
dividuation is being expressed in growth and physico-chemical
reactions. When form and bodily function have become so well
integrated that the organism can act as a unit *vis-à-vis* the world,
mental reactions appear. These for a long evolutionary period

are, apparently, simple and so relatively small in number that their combinations are few and stable (simple instincts). Gradually, however, the range of reactions increases and with this the complexity of combinations, which means an increased modifiability of patterns. Finally, a self-determination on the psychological level appears and this is consciousness. At this point, the patterns are incredibly complicated, and have attained such facility in composition and decomposition that human mental reactions may change and new ones appear every second. According to this scheme, the same principles apply in the formation of an atom as apply to the creation of consciousness, and at every stage the directing agencies are immaterial.

At this point, one important corollary should be considered. It might be said that, if these patterns are immaterial, and if, at the conscious mental level, they can be controlled by the super-pattern consciousness, this would open the door to magic and give every conscious being supernatural powers. The corollary answers this objection, and indeed, shows how magic is impossible. In the hierarchy of patterns, control exerted by any pattern is only over the elements integrated to form that pattern: the element is treated as a unit and, indeed, the pattern is concerned only with the properties of the units and not with the lower level components which may have, in turn, been integrated to form the units. A formula may make this clearer. If α, β, γ, etc. are integrated to form the pattern a, and if a be integrated with b and c to form A, then A controls a, b and c but has no direct influence over α, β, or γ. Indirectly, of course, it may succeed in activating α, β, or γ, but only in virtue of having aroused a. For instance, I cannot by any direct volition succeed in producing an extra secretion of adrenalin. But I can produce it indirectly by willing excessive muscular exertion which, in turn, activates a complex of sympathetic nervous system functions among which is adrenal secretion. If I cannot produce a simple physiological change selectively, how much less could I, by mere willing it, affect the inorganic world? Since magic has become a term of abuse that is substituted for argument, it may be well to state what I mean by it. Magic, I take it, is the production of effects not predictable, nor thinkable, as a result of the manipulation of the materials used, which operate according to the known laws of the properties of those materials. If the pattern theory be sound, much of so-called science is magical, as, for instance, when it attempts to account for mind in terms of physics and chemistry. Similarly, the doctrine of transubstantiation, when defined as a spiritual phenomenon is not magic, because the manipulations are symbolic. Psychology cannot now (and may very well never be able to) discuss spiritual phenomena, except as emotional states. We know, however, that all the finer emotions are mediated by symbolic words and actions; so there is nothing magical about a ritual use of bread and wine giving a feeling of the Real Presence.[1]

Some time after the pattern metaphysic had reached in my mind the form that is outlined above, Whitehead's book *Science and the Modern World* appeared. I was greatly surprised on reading it to find that, proceeding from the level of mathematical physics, Whitehead had apparently arrived at much the same general formulations about Nature as I had done. Unfortunately, I am unfamiliar with mathematical reasoning, and its terms may have different meanings from those which the same words carry in daily speech. Consequently, I cannot be confident that my scheme really is the same as his. Perhaps readers disciplined in natural philosophy may be able to judge as to the similarity of our views from the following quotation:

"The atomic material entities which are considered in physical science are merely these individual enduring entities, conceived in abstraction from everything except what concerns their mutual interplay in determining each other's historical routes of life-history. Such entities are partially formed by the inheritance of aspects from their own past.

[1] It should be admitted that there is an exception—perhaps only an apparent one—to the statement that consciousness cannot effect simple physiological changes selectively. A phenomenon of this order does occur in hysteria and may be experimentally produced under hypnosis in favourable subjects. Isolated portions of the gastro-intestinal tract may shew paralysis or over-activity and, at the surface of the body, inflammatory changes can be varied in extent and in time of healing, even if they cannot be produced without any actual irritation. (The evidence for the last is unsatisfactory, as the investigators who claim it have not taken adequate precautions to prevent the subjects wounding themselves surreptitiously.) It would seem that, in these cases, there is an unconscious control of isolated bodily functions, analogous to that of consciousness over the movement of one finger independently of its fellows, although the former functions seem, normally, to be regulated by patterns of a physiological and inframental order. A proper discussion of the general problem thus raised is impossible at this point, for it involves principles displayed best in the functions of consciousness and must, therefore, be postponed to another volume. I may say now, however, that there are reasons for considering, on the one hand, that the hysterical and hypnotic phenomena are pathological and, on the other, that they may serve as one of the points of departure in a programme of rationalizing the "supernatural", which is not merely cheap magic. Unsatisfactory though it may be to leave such an important problem in the air, it would be idle to discuss it in the absence of a mass of pertinent data.

But they are also partially formed by the aspects of other events forming their environments. The laws of physics are the laws declaring how the entities mutually react among themselves. For physics these laws are arbitrary, because that science has abstracted from what the entities are in themselves. We have seen that this fact of what the entities are in themselves is liable to modification by their environments. Accordingly, the assumption that no modification of these laws is to be looked for in environments, which have any striking difference from the environments for which the laws have been observed to hold, is very unsafe. The physical entities may be modified in very essential ways, so far as these laws are concerned. It is even possible that they may be developed into individualities of more fundamental types, with wider embodiment of envisagement. Such envisagement might reach to the attainment of the poising of alternative values with exercise of choice lying outside the physical laws, and expressible only in terms of purpose. Apart from such remote possibilities, it remains an immediate deduction than an individual entity, whose own life-history is a part within the life-history of some larger, deeper, more complete pattern, is liable to have aspects of that larger pattern dominating its own being, and to experience modifications of that larger pattern reflected in itself as modifications of its own being. This is the theory of organic mechanism."[1]

I have been asked the question: What is the relation between "patterns" and "laws"? "Law" is defined in the *New English Dictionary* as follows: "In the sciences of observation, a theoretical principle deduced from particular facts, applicable to a defined group or class of phenomena and expressible by the statement that a particular phenomenon always occurs if certain conditions be present. In the physical sciences, and occasionally in others, called more explicitly *law of nature*, or *natural law*". This is perhaps equivalent to saying that a law is a descriptive generalization about facts carrying with it a prediction as to the repetition of the phenomena. If insistence be made on the "always occurs", it could, of course, be argued that certainty as to the validity of any natural law is impossible. The discovery of radio-activity and the observations from which the theory of relativity began unsettled a number of laws previously regarded as having universal application. The only safe statement, in any given case, is that there is a tendency for the particular phenomenon to recur when its conditions, as set forth in the law, are present, although presumably the predictability would be absolute, if *all* the conditions were known. The definition gives to a law more than mere description when it introduces this element of prediction. This implies the existence of a process, a dynamic something, which produces the pheno-

_____
[1] *Loc. cit.* pp. 150–1.

menon. In a pattern this second element is accentuated. It might
be held that a law merely describes the conditions producing a
phenomenon, and states that these conditions are the cause of the
phenomenon. If this be so, a law is wholly inert and its difference
from a pattern can be stated clearly. For a pattern is not a description of causes and results, it is that which unites them: it is the
process itself. It is a law which has become dynamic and is responsible for the sequence of the events which it correlates.

This seems to be the function of the formulae with which
physicists are now working. In the biological world (including
the psychological), there are two conditions for the expression of a
pattern. The first is that structures be present, which are suitable
for the exercise of the correlated functions, or at least be sufficiently
represented to make possible an expression of the relation in
question. The second is that a suitable stimulus be present: the
stimulus is one of the elements integrated in the pattern, or some
representation thereof. It usually originates in an environmental
event, but may be an internal visceral disturbance or an imaginal
process. At the conscious psychological level, the stimulus may be
a goal for a programme of actions, and it seems probable that
purpose may act similarly in evolution and in individual development. Whether a pattern is always activated when these general
conditions are fulfilled is a question impossible to answer in the
present state of our knowledge, but I may mention a few phenomena, otherwise inexplicable, which might be explained on this basis.

In the biological field there is the puzzling phenomenon known
as convergent evolution. Two species or genera of plants or animals
may shew extraordinary resemblance, although it is clear that they
are not blood-relatives, so to speak, having had quite different
ancestry. An excellent example is the occurrence in Australasia
of animals that have the general form and habits of the cat and
dog tribes we are familiar with, although they belong to a separate
section of the general mammalian stock. A wolf is more closely
related to a whale than to the Australasian thylacine, yet the un-
sophisticated would mistake the latter for a wolf. Examples of
such convergence go clean beyond the range of coincidence and
make the assumption of purpose in evolution difficult to avoid.
(Materialistic biologists are prone to leave such phenomena alone
in their general formulations.) The pattern hypothesis, however,
provides a ready explanation for convergent evolution. The "dog"
pattern being once firmly established, it will tend to recur when-

ever conditions and habit of life make the canine type of adaptation expedient and the stock has structures and functions that can be utilized for the expression of the pattern.

In the psychological field we are confronted with the alleged occurrence of the same idea in people who are not in apparent communication with one another, and with the undoubted phenomenon of the transmission of ideas from individual to individual without adequate means of communication, or at least, without there being any conscious knowledge of the mode of transmission. The latter group is easier to deal with, so we may begin with it. This is the phenomenon of intuition and is seen most clearly in group behaviour. Observe, for instance, the variations in the flight of a flock of birds. They fly swiftly forward and then suddenly wheel, without the observer being able to detect the passage of the signal from one bird to another: they seem to act as a unit and not as individuals. This is, presumably, more than mere semblance. There is a group pattern which lowers the threshold for stimuli arising in the group to such a point that apparent unanimity is achieved. Were the threshold lowered to zero, there would then be true telepathy and an individual bird would respond in concert with the others, even though it were cut off from visual and auditory connection with them. So far as I know, there is no evidence of this, so we may presume that the individual patterns have merely a very low threshold, because the group pattern, which is constituted of their integration, is in activity. In favour of this view is the fact that the attention of the individual bird is deflected from the environment, which would be one indication of attention being given to the group. The following is an example of this. When driving a car, I have countless times seen a bird flying straight for the windscreen and have expected to see it dashed to pieces. Always, at the last instant, the bird swerves. Once, however, it did happen. A flock of starlings was flying in an opposite direction to that of my path and an outlying one, flying straight at the car for a distance of at least fifty feet, made no effort whatever to swerve and was, of course, killed instantly.

A similar phenomenon appears in the almost synchronous change of behaviour in the members of a human mob and in the spread of rumour. In both these instances, however, it is easy to detect the presence of the stimulus which excites the reaction in each individual. But, in order to have the stimulus of this strength effective, a group activity, to which it is pertinent, must be in progress. Rumour, for instance, will spread like wild-fire when a country is at war, or an important election is imminent, although the individuals who transmit it would pay no attention to the story in question under other circumstances. Similar mechanisms probably operate between two individuals who are said to read each other's minds. What usually happens is that they are in sympathy one with another: this implies that they have many meanings in common and that the same stimulus will, therefore, produce analogous reactions, which are largely emotional. The ideas that emerge to consciousness are more apt to be merely similar than identical, although the desire for unanimity will be likely to make one or the other modify the conscious formation, until it coincides literally with that of the other. Each is then satisfied that identical ideas have originated synchronously. Morton Prince has done excellent work in demonstrating that many "occult" phenomena have originated in perceptions that were not consciously registered, but were received and elaborated unconsciously, and then emerged in consciousness or behaviour as the apparent product of telepathy or spiritistic control.

If true telepathy exists it must be a case, in our terminology, of the threshold for communication being lowered to zero. If the conditions under which this might occur be explained, we may then judge as to whether it is likely to happen or not. Any given reaction appears as the result of an actual environmental stimulus, or as part of the activity of an interest of which it is a component part. In the present case, the actual stimulus would be direct communication, which is totally absent if true telepathy occurred. The secondary excitation of the specific pattern must, therefore, be as one exhibition of an interest. If two persons are closely associated for years and in sympathy, they may, by mutual influence, develop similar interests, although never identical ones. Interests, in turn, are activated by environmental events, including visceral disturbances *via* appetites, or by personality, which is an integration of interests. So far as the activation of interests is concerned, our case again eliminates the environmental stimulus, leaving only the personality influence. Again it is conceivable, although less likely, that two persons could have similar personalities. Let us now see what the chances are of telepathy being explained on a pattern basis. An individual *A* has a given experience *X*, which *B* is also to experience, although in a totally separate environment. *X* arouses an interest important for *A* and orients his personality in a given direction, of which X and its reaction are but one expression. According to the general conditions laid down above for the activation of patterns, a well integrated pattern may find a substitutive expression in another organism provided the second organism is potentially capable of it and it fits in with the general trend of the latter's behaviour. But this is only likely to occur when the pattern is pre-potent as a result of many repetitions. It is conceivable that X might cause the establishment of such a pattern in A if he were sensitized for that kind of experience, but this would probably only eventuate following a long rumination after the event. Presuming, however, that it does happen immediately, B's personality might be affected, and shew a sudden activation of the interest in question. For the telepathic communication to be transmitted *via* patterns it is now necessary that, as an apparent stimulus for this interest in B's mind, the experience X should be imaged. That this could happen must be admitted, but it would be a matter of coincidence, for there is nothing in our laws of patterns to make probable the imaginal reproduction by an interest of one stimulus rather than another from among the group that have been conditioned therewith. At each step, the telepathy seems unlikely with accumulative improbability. All that "patterns" could do would be to limit the range within which coincidence operated.

For more than a score of years, I have been interested in this problem and have, therefore, made a note of every occurrence in myself of an apparently telepathic message. Many a time I have been overtaken by the conviction that some accident had befallen a friend or relative, but on making enquiry I have never been able to discover the slightest actual cause for my misgiving. Consequently, if I should now get news of some mishap to a friend, concerning whom I had been anxious, I should be inclined to regard the phenomenon as one of coincidence. But such a coincidence twenty years ago might have made me a believer in telepathy. The patterns which are the essence of thoughts are certainly immaterial, and telepathy (if it exists) must be a transmission of something immaterial. But the former cannot be invoked to explain the latter, unless there be patterns of a super-psychological character of which we know nothing as yet. If such there be, we shall be entitled to assume them only when a sufficiently extensive body of "psychic" data have been collected to enable us to formulate laws as to their occurrence. And that day is far distant. I must hasten to add, however, that, though patterns may explain many of the rules by which natural phenomena are governed, it would be foolish to say that they explain the universe.

It is a big enough problem to analyse the causes of the phenomena that bombard our senses daily, and it is one on which we have only begun. It is conceivable, however, that if the shackles of materialism are thrown off, we may move more quickly on our quest than has recently been possible. Materialistic zeal has lead to the acquisition of an enormous mass of facts, and science has more pabulum to-day than it can digest. It is time to sit down and think. Fortunately, some physicists are doing so, as the following words shew: "Eddington hints that a real law of nature is likely to stand out by the fact that it appears to us irrational, since in that case it is less likely that we have invented it to satisfy our intellectual taste. And from this point of view he inclines to the belief that the quantum-principle is the first real law of nature that has been discovered in physics".[1]

This statement, reminiscent of the theologian's *Credo quia impossibile*, may, perhaps, foreshadow an enormous and revolutionary change in the human mind. If the concept be once established that relations, rather than direct sensory experience, are fundamental, then values, previously relegated to religion and art, will become commonplace and paramount in greatly enriched lives. That for which the human spirit yearns will become "scientific". This is not an impossible development, for we have hardly outgrown animism and we should be able to recapture and nurture the truth that is in it. Animism, which is a child's philosophy, may be defined as a recognition of patterns which are distorted into demonology. That is, the patterns are personified, and then attention is deflected to their imaginary human attributes. In our revolt against superstition we have, as Eddington hints, become sterile in our rationality. Ordinary present day intelligence is fearful of what cannot be grasped consciously and formulated in terms of the obvious and palpable. So intuition is taboo. Every original scientist thinks first in "pattern" concepts, but, like Darwin, he leaves his inspired thoughts in his notes, and gives the world an argument which is, psychologically, only a rationalization. Should relationships, however, become more "real" than the phenomena they govern, then intuition would come into its own.

[1] Bertrand Russell, *loc. cit.* p. 170.

INDEX

For EU product safety concerns, contact us at Calle de José Abascal, 56–1°,
28003 Madrid, Spain or eugpsr@cambridge.org.

www.ingramcontent.com/pod-product-compliance
Ingram Content Group UK Ltd.
Pitfield, Milton Keynes, MK11 3LW, UK
UKHW030859150625
459647UK00021B/2724